Philosophy of Psychopharmacology

Philosophy of Psychopharmacology

Smart Pills, Happy Pills, and Pepp Pills

Dan J. Stein, M.D., Ph.D., D.Phil.

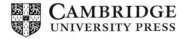

CAMBRIDGE
UNIVERSITY PRESS

CAMBRIDGE UNIVERSITY PRESS
Cambridge, New York, Melbourne, Madrid, Cape Town, Singapore, São Paulo, Delhi

Cambridge University Press
The Edinburgh Building, Cambridge CB2 8RU, UK

Published in the United States of America by Cambridge University Press, New York

www.cambridge.org
Information on this title: www.cambridge.org/9780521856522

First published 2008

Printed in the United Kingdom at the University Press, Cambridge

A catalogue record for this publication is available from the British Library

Library of Congress Cataloguing in Publication data

Stein, Dan J.
    Smart pills, happy pills, pepp pills : philosophy of psychopharmacology / Dan J. Stein.
        p. ; cm.
    Includes bibliographical references and index.
    ISBN 978-0-521-85652-2 (hardback)
    1. Psychopharmacology–Philosophy.   2. Psychotropic drugs.   3. Psychotherapy.   I. Title.
    [DNLM: 1. Psychopharmacology.   2. Brain–drug effects.   3. Mental Disorders–drug
    therapy.   4. Philosophy, Medical.   5. Psychotropic Drugs.   QV 77 S819s 2008]

    RM315.S886   2008
    615'.78 – dc22   2008021912

ISBN 978-0-521-85652-2 hardback

Contents

Preface

At times, new scientific data lead to a revolution in how we think about ourselves. Copernicus's data showed that the Earth and its inhabitants were not situated at the geographic epicentre of the Universe. Darwin's observations indicated that humans did not exist in a natural realm apart from other primates. Freud's cases suggested that the rational conscious mind was not necessarily the primary determinant of human behaviour. This volume begins with the idea that revolutionary data about the brain and the mind, and especially about medications that act on the brain-mind, will fundamentally change our thoughts about humans.

Brain-mind-altering or psychoactive substances, also known as psychotropics, have been used since antiquity for both recreational and therapeutic reasons. Noah celebrated with wine, and Plato philosophized about its appropriate use.[1] Paracelsus knew the value of laudanum, and Pinel not only unshackled the insane but also prescribed opium. Nevertheless, the modern field of empirical psychopharmacology is only a few decades old. Psychopharmacologists have mostly been interested in basic science investigations of the mechanism of new drugs and in clinical studies of their efficacy in treating psychiatric disorders. They have not paid much attention to the more abstract question of whether their data change our understanding of the nature of cognitive science and of psychiatry. This is an important gap, and this volume hopes to begin to close it.

Working with the new psychiatric drugs raises crucial philosophical questions, and so encourages a rethinking of cognitive science and particularly of psychiatry. The value of the new psychiatric drugs as

---

[1] Plato's "A Touchstone for Courage" (Plato, 1970) is perhaps the first philosophy of psychopharmacology in the West. Aristotle similarly considered issues around alcohol and responsibility (Aristotle, 1980).

things-with-which-to-think (Papert, 1980) lies not only in their efficacy for major psychiatric disorders, but also in their potential use in
a range of additional contexts. There is, for example, growing interest
in smart drugs to improve intellectual, sporting, or military performance, in mood-brightening and personality-enhancing drugs, and
in pep pills to enhance motivation and energy. Scientists and societies are increasingly grappling with questions about using medical
treatments, including psychotropics, for purposes that are "Beyond
Therapy" (President's Council on Bioethics, 2003), or "Better than
Well" (Elliott, 2003).

Such so-called "cosmetic psychopharmacology" (Kramer, 1997)
immediately raises a range of conceptual (or metaphysical) questions
about the nature of the entities that are used by psychiatrists: How do we
best define medical and psychiatric disorders? Are psychiatric disorders
a kind of medical disorder, or are they a different kind of category? Can
psychotropics change personality, and if so, what are the implications
for our concepts of self? How do we distinguish the use of psychotropics
for therapy from their use for enhancement, or psychotropic medications from legal substances such as alcohol, illicit substances such as
cocaine, and nutrients or nutraceuticals?

Second, psychopharmacological data raise a series of explanatory (or
epistemological) questions focused on how to best understand brain-
behaviour phenomena. How can we understand the way in which psychotropics work to alter thoughts, feelings, and behaviours, and should
our explanations differ from those we develop for understanding how
psychotherapy leads to change? How can we best conceptualize placebo
and nocebo responses to psychotropics, and the relevant unconscious
processes involved? What is the relevance of Darwinian or evolutionary
mechanisms when investigating psychopharmacological phenomena?

Third, psychopharmacological data raise a series of moral (or ethical)
questions. When is the use of psychotropics for psychiatric disorders
appropriate? Depressive realism refers to the phenomenon that people
with depression appear to be more realistic in their appraisals of the
world, the self, and the future than are people without depression –
is depressive realism best left untreated? Should cosmetic psychopharmacology – the treatment of undesirable traits (poor memory, shyness,

impulsivity) that cannot be characterized as psychiatric disorders – be encouraged or deplored, do we believe in a pill for every psychic ill?

To discuss the questions raised by psychopharmacology, we need a framework that can address related questions in philosophy of science, medicine, language, mind, emotion, personal identity, the unconscious, and evolution. I have found it useful to summarize this immense philosophical literature by contrasting two camps – a "*classical*" and a "*critical*" approach to cognitive and clinical science. While this contrast entails a great deal of oversimplification, and may not apply to the work of any particular thinker, it serves as a useful foundation for putting forward an integrative approach to answering the questions of psychopharmacology.

Very briefly, the classical position can be traced back to Plato, runs through the work of the early Wittgenstein, was taken up by the logical positivists, and continues to be a major force in contemporary philosophy. It has viewed cognition in terms of computation, and has defined psychiatric disorders in similarly restrictive ways. In contrast, the critical position also has early roots, was strongly influenced by thinkers like Vico and Herder, played an important role in post-modern movements, and continues to be central for continental philosophy. It has emphasized the importance of human understanding and of social context, and has regarded mental disorders as representing merely another way of living.

Instead, this volume puts forward an approach that highlights the findings of cognitive-affective science; this is a framework that allows for an approach to the brain-mind that emphasizes the embodiment of cognition and affect in neuronal circuitry and in the interaction of people with the physical and social world, and that provides an expansive space for considering psychiatric disorders as complex, significant, and real phenomena. It is an approach that is consistent with a naturalized philosophy, with scientific realism, and also with a range of psychological and philosophical work that views the brain-mind as neither a computational algorithm, nor as a social construct, but rather as fundamentally embodied.

The term "cognitive-affective" is used here rather than merely "cognitive" or "affective", because the affective realm and its integration with the cognitive one has been too-often ignored in both psychology and philosophy of psychology. The term "brain-mind" is used rather than merely "brain" or "mind", again to emphasize how the two constructs are, in fact, impossible to disentangle. Similarly, I later refer to "psychobiological" mechanisms. These hyphenated constructs, although perhaps clumsy at first, serve to highlight, first, how complex thoughts and feelings are ultimately based in more basic constructs such as body representation, and second, how the brain-mind is not a computational apart-from-the-world passive reflector, but rather a thinking-feeling actor-in-the-world and active constructor.

Psychotropics are remarkably useful things with-which-to-think. This is not only because they are used in a range of different contexts, but also because of the highly complex issues that they raise, touching on questions in philosophy of science, medicine, language, mind, emotion, personal identity, the unconscious, and evolution. Conversely, answers to the questions raised by advances in psychopharmacology may have profound implications for a broad range of philosophical problems, including metaphysical, epistemological, and moral issues. Wittgenstein was fond of the metaphor of philosophy as a useful medical treatment; this volume suggests that psychopharmacology provides a useful subject matter for philosophy.[2]

Insofar as this volume addresses so many well-discussed questions in philosophy, much of it depends on standing on the shoulders of giants. I am particularly indebted to the work of Roy Bhaskar on philosophy of science, George Lakoff on the cognitive science of categories, and Mark Johnson on moral reasoning. Arguments here are informed by a broad range of philosophical work, including writings at the intersection of philosophy and psychiatry – pioneered by Karl Jaspers, and now an increasingly productive area.

At the same time, I would venture that comparatively little philosophical work has been done in the area of psychopharmacology in

---

[2] The work of a number of important physician-philosophers, such as William James and Karl Jaspers, begins with a careful consideration of psychology and psychopathology. Subsequently, a number of philosophers such as Austin (in the linguistic-analytic tradition) and Merleau-Ponty (in the continental tradition) early on suggested or employed psychiatry as a significant resource for philosophy.

general, and cosmetic psychopharmacology in particular. This volume outlines philosophical questions raised by psychopharmacology, discusses possible answers from the classical and critical perspectives, and draws on the cognitive-affective sciences to provide an integrated set of answers. I hope that by doing so, the volume contributes to providing a conceptual foundation for good clinical psychopharmacology.

Solomon Stein gave me a life-long interest in the question of whether pharmacology was good or bad. Sally and Leslie Swartz were instrumental in helping me to begin on the road to philosophy more than two decades ago. Jeremy Barris, Arnold Abramovitz, Ronald Rieder, and Michael Schwartz gave encouragement at crucial points. Derek Bolton helped give me the courage to pursue the current project. Anton van Niekerk was crucial in providing a supportive intellectual framework within which I could attempt to move forward. Both Derek and Anton gave me a great deal of encouragement, as well as many useful comments on drafts of the manuscript; this work would not have appeared without their generous mentorship. Many other colleagues have helped me think through questions covered here; particular thanks to Ineke Bolt, George Ellis, Jacques Kriel, Wittem Landman, Ronald Pies, and Willem David Walywn for their comments and suggestions on early versions. Finally, I wish to acknowledge with deep gratitude my wife, Heather, and my children, Gabriella, Joshua, and Sarah, who have put up with my irritable mood when attempting to do philosophy, as well as with the inevitable absences from family life that this attempt entailed.

Psychopharmacology – a remarkable development

Psychopharmacology, the study of psychotropics, or brain-mind-altering substances, is a fascinating field at the confluence of neurochemistry and behaviour. Basic psychopharmacologists are mostly interested in how psychotropics work, often studying neurochemical properties of different compounds in animal models. Clinical psychopharmacologists are mainly interested in the clinical applications of psychotropics, often working in psychiatric settings. But what exactly are psychotropics? How in fact do they work? How widely are they used, and do they really help people?

In this chapter I begin by outlining the broad scope of psychopharmacology: emphasizing that psychotropics have been long, widely, and intensively used by humankind for a range of purposes; describing the relatively recent birth of modern psychopharmacology as an empirical science; and noting that despite the remarkable progress in the field to date, psychopharmacology is at an early stage in its development. Then, in the next chapter I go on to consider the major philosophical issues raised by the advent of modern psychopharmacology.

The length, breadth, and depth of psychotropic use

And he drank of the wine, and was drunken; and he was uncovered within his tent. (Genesis 9:21, King James Version)

What is better adapted than the festive use of wine, in the first place to test, and in the second place to train the character of a man, if care be taken in the use of it? (Plato, 1970)

Humans use psychotropic agents in a range of different contexts. We imbibe stimulants such as caffeine as part of our regular diet and to enhance our attention and performance, we celebrate social occasions and perform religious rites with alcohol, we experiment with consciousness-altering drugs, and we take psychiatric medications when we suffer from symptoms such as depression and anxiety. There is no reason to suspect that we have not been engaged in these kinds of activities since the dawn of human time (Moreno, 2006a; Playfair, 1987; Rivers, 2001).

This use of psychotropic agents by *Homo sapiens* is remarkable in a number of different ways. For one thing, reliance on psychotropics is a phenomenon that differentiates humankind from most other species. In the laboratory, a range of animals can certainly become addicted to substances. But in the wild, there is only accidental contact with psychotropics. While there have been occasional reports of non-human primate use of plants for medicinal purposes, such reports have rarely if ever extended to psychotropic agents (Rodriguez *et al.*, 1985; Whiten & Boesch, 2001).

Indeed, in comparison to the use of other pharmaceuticals, human use of psychotropics is remarkable for its broad range. Humans throughout the world have long relied on agents that act on organs such as the gut, the skin, or the heart. However, such pharmaceuticals have invariably been restricted to the prevention or treatment of symptoms of disorders. In contrast, psychotropics have a range of other uses, including as an everyday nutrient and social "lubricant" (spirits), a component of religious rituals and spiritual voyages (entheogens), and performance or cognitive enhancers (nootropics).

The use of psychotropics is also notable for its intensiveness. Ginseng, for example, is a psychotropic herb that played a key role in changing the fortune of Chinese dynasties, due to its high demand and the consequent profits earned from its trade (Taylor, 2006). Alcohol, opium, and cocaine are amongst the addictive substances that have been at the centre of underground battles or international wars, again because each has a substantial market. Modern psychotropic medications have been blockbusters for the pharmaceutical industry, earning it billions of dollars in revenue.

This broad and deep range of uses depends in turn on the complexity of our nervous system – which provides multiple targets for psychotropics to act on, and on the importance of this system to our being – so that psychotropics can have wide-ranging and profound effects. It also reflects the vast range of psychotropics available to our species; psychoactive agents are found in abundance in the plant kingdom (e.g. steroidal hormones are found in yams, monoamine oxidase inhibitors are present in St John's wort, alcohol is obtainable from fermented fruits), and are now also readily synthesized in the laboratory.

Pharmacological agents may in general be the same as endogenous compounds (e.g. insulin for diabetes), may act as agonists or antagonists at particular receptors so augmenting or blocking endogenous processes (e.g. diuretics enhance diuresis), or may have complex stabilizing or destabilizing effects (e.g. anticonvulsants lower seizure threshold). In the case of psychotropics, we have agents that employ each of these possibilities (e.g. exogenous testosterone acts in the same way as endogenous testosterone, selective serotonin reuptake inhibitors enhance serotonergic neurotransmission, alcohol has destabilizing effects on neuronal membranes).

The advent of empirical psychopharmacology

He who had drunk of this potion would not shed tears for a whole day even if his mother and his father were to die, and even if his most beloved son were slaughtered before his eyes. (Homer, *Odyssey*)

Psychopharmacology is an interdisciplinary science in which many techniques and branches of knowledge are brought together. In seeking to modify human behaviour by the use of chemical substances, it lies at the crossroads of the biological sciences and the humanities, because every psychopharmacological problem concerns the relationship between the body and the mind. (Delay, 2006)

The history of psychopharmacology is notable for its length and breadth and depth, but the advent of psychopharmacology as an empirical science is a recent development (Healy, 2002). The term "psychopharmacology" has been in use since the early twentieth century, and gained currency in the 1950s, at a time when the first randomized controlled trials of psychotropic agents were undertaken (Thullier, 1999).[1] The field grew exponentially thereafter, driven by rapid advances in both basic science (e.g. molecular neurobiology, behavioural pharmacology, synthetic chemistry) and in clinical science (e.g. operational diagnosis, symptom measurement, trials methodology).

First-generation psychotropics were often found serendipitously. For example, the first antipsychotic agent, chlorpromazine, was developed as an anaesthetic; when it was later found to decrease psychotic symptoms, further investigation established that it was a dopamine blocker (Thullier, 1999). Similarly, the first monoamine oxidase inhibitor – a powerful class of antidepressants – was developed as an antituberculous drug. Once again, investigation of the mechanisms of action led to a focus on monoamines in depression.

Whereas these early agents often had multiple actions, affecting different receptors, second-generation agents were specifically developed in order to act on one receptor at a time. A well-known example is fluoxetine, originally marketed as Prozac, a selective serotonin reuptake inhibitor (or SSRI). In contrast to the tricyclic antidepressant agents, which act on serotonin and noradrenaline receptors, as well as on the cholinergic system, fluoxetine primarily affects the serotonin system. Interestingly, recent agents have been specifically engineered to act on more than one receptor system. These potentially offer the advantage of altering the multiple neurotransmitter systems that may be involved in complex disorders.

A number of points can be made about modern psychotropics. First, they cannot be likened to neuronal sledgehammers – fluoxetine acts on the product of a single gene (of the 23 000 odd in the human body). Second, their effects are nevertheless complex – serotonin interacts with multiple other systems, so that fluoxetine eventually affects a

---

[1] One of the first to use the term "psychopharmacology" was Jean Delay, a pioneering French psychiatrist who testified in the Nuremberg trials and who had a doctorate in philosophy. During the student protests of 1968, strongly influenced by the work of psychiatrists or those using examples from psychiatry (Fanon, Foucault, Goffman, Laing, Marcuse, Szasz), his office was ransacked, and he was forced to resign.

range of neuronal circuits and ultimately thoughts and emotions and behaviours. Most psychotropics can be termed neuromodulators – they act on multiple circuits that spread throughout the brain. Third, the adverse effects of psychotropics are sometimes overstated; for example, while some medications are addicting, antipsychotics and antidepressants are not. Fourth, this does not mean they do not have crucially important side effects – they do.

Progress in psychopharmacology has had an enormous influence on the theory and practice of psychiatry. Indeed, psychiatry is now primarily "biological" in its approach – whereas the field (particularly in the USA) was dominated by psychoanalytic theories and practices in the 1950s, by the end of the twentieth century psychiatric research leaned strongly on the neurosciences, and psychiatric practice relied heavily on psychopharmacological interventions (Luhrmann, 2000; Sabshin, 1990; Shorter, 1998). While psychiatrists continue to be trained in psychotherapy, and optimal prescription of psychotropics requires a rigorous appreciation of the psychodynamics of the patient, the shift in the field has been revolutionary in its extent and impact.

These developments need to be understood not only in terms of the scientific advances allowed by the new psychotropics, but also in more socio-political terms. The pharmaceutical industry has played a key role in developing and marketing psychotropic products (Angell, 2004; Degrandpre, 2006; Healy, 2004; McHenry, 2006; Moynihan & Smith, 2002; Smith, 1991; Starcevic, 2002; Szasz, 2001; Valenstein, 1998). Although much research on psychopharmacology is funded by government sources, such as the National Institutes of Health in the USA, most large, randomized, controlled trials on psychotropics are funded by the industry. Indeed, psychotropics have proven to be particularly profitable pharmaceutical agents; the market for these agents amounts to billions of dollars per annum (IMS Health, 2002). Large amounts of money may be devoted even to niche areas, such as work on psychotropics to enhance performance in the military (Moreno, 2006b).

The relationship between academic psychopharmacology and the pharmaceutical industry has been subjected to a number of critiques. There are, for example, important concerns about the objectivity of academic researchers who are primarily funded by industry (Angell, 2004; Healy, 2004). Clinicians have in turn been criticized for over-diagnosing and overtreating psychiatric disorders (Horwitz & Wakefield, 2007; Moynihan & Smith, 2002). More radically, an antipsychiatry movement, which questions the scientific validity of psychiatric diagnoses, and is concerned that psychiatric interventions are better understood in terms of the control of social deviance, has criticised the use of "chemical straitjackets" and the marketing of psychotropics as panaceas (Breggin, 1993; Ingleby, 1981; Sedgwick, 1982).

Gains and gaps in psychopharmacology

The expectations I have formulated some 25 years ago regarding developments in the pharmacotherapy of depression have not, or only to a small extent, materialized. Neither have they been refuted. (van Praag, 2001)

Critiques of psychopharmacology which emphasize the use of medication to control social deviance, and criticize the use of "chemical straitjackets" and the marketing of psychotropics as panaceas, ignore some empirical data. First, the global burden of psychiatric disorder is enormous, with 5 of the 10 most disabling medical disorders comprising neuropsychiatric conditions (Murray & Lopez, 1996), and second, despite their prevalence and associated impairment, severe psychiatric disorders continue to remain relatively underdiagnosed and under-treated in both developed and developing countries (Demyttenaere et al., 2004). Nevertheless, this volume is primarily concerned with potential problems in the widespread use of psychotropic agents for a range of other psychic ills. While there may have been major gains in psychopharmacology, it is important to also understand the significant gaps in this field.

Modern psychopharmacology has on the one hand arguably achieved remarkable successes. The closure of large, long-term psychiatric hospitals – deinstitutionalization – was largely brought about by the success of antipsychotic agents in treating serious psychotic disorders such as schizophrenia and bipolar disorder. Although depression and anxiety disorders continue to be underdiagnosed and undertreated, there are now effective medications available for many psychiatric conditions. Although not all data are consistent (Helgason *et al.*, 2004), it is possible that decreases in the prevalence of suicide in some developed countries reflect the better diagnosis and pharmacotherapy of depression (Carlsten *et al.*, 2001).

Modern antipsychotics and antidepressants are relatively safe, well-tolerated, and non-addicting, so that many early concerns about the use of psychotropic agents for psychiatric disorders have diminished over time. New psychotropics are introduced only after carefully conducted randomized controlled trials show both safety and efficacy. The pharmaceutical industry is closely regulated by governmental agencies. Advances in basic mechanisms continue to be made, new agents continue to be introduced, and there is no reason not to suspect that future pharmacological interventions will be even more useful than those currently available.

At the same time, there are notable gaps in our knowledge of the brain-mind in general (Sala, 1999), and of psychopharmacology in particular. First, a full appreciation of the mechanisms of action of psychotropics remains a goal for the future. Although we understand a good deal about the receptors at which most psychotropics act, we understand much less about how changes at these receptors translate into further changes "downstream" at the so-called 2nd and 3rd messenger level, and we do not have a complete understanding of how these changes in turn alter systems that underpin cognition and affect.

Furthermore, currently available psychotropics almost all work by changing monoaminergic neurotransmitter systems; despite the introduction of new and useful drugs in recent decades, these continue to work on similar pathways as did the earliest agents. Thus, although many psychopharmacologists are excited about the progress that has occurred, a number have warned against exaggerating what has been achieved (van Praag, 1998). While modern agents may be better tolerated than older ones, the lack of truly innovative new interventions in psychopharmacology is worrisome to many.

An early idea in psychopharmacology was that of "pharmacotherapeutic dissection"; if disorders A and B responded to medication X but not Y, while disorders C and D responded to medication Y but not to X – then disorders A and B would have nosological and biological overlap with one another, but not with the overlapping disorders C and D (Klein, 1964). Obsessive–compulsive disorder (OCD), for example, responds more robustly to clomipramine, a predominantly serotoninergic re-uptake inhibitor, than to desipramine, an agent that is also a tricyclic antidepressant, but that is predominantly a noradrenergic reuptake inhibitor (Zohar *et al.*, 1988). Furthermore, benzodiazepines are useful in certain anxiety disorders, but not in OCD. Analogously, whereas dopamine blockers typically cause sedation in healthy volunteers, they result in a decrease in psychotic symptoms in those with schizophrenia or bipolar disorder, underscoring the boundaries between psychotic disorders and normality.

Nevertheless, this principle has not been entirely productive in more contemporary research; for example, clomipramine is more effective than desipramine not only for a number of conditions that have much in common with obsessive–compulsive disorder (e.g. body dysmorphic disorder), but also for a number of apparently quite unrelated conditions (e.g. premenstrual dysphoric disorder) (Stein, 2001). Conversely, when a medication is effective, we cannot necessarily deduce a great deal about the mechanisms involved in the relevant disorder. It turns out that there is surprisingly little evidence of serotonergic dysfunction per se in OCD. It is possible that a quite different neurochemical system is at fault in OCD, and that serotonergic medications are effective only via their secondary effects on that other system (Stein, 2002). Furthermore, dopamine-releasing agents are not only effective in improving concentrations in patients diagnosed with attention-deficit/hyperactivity disorder (AD/HD), they may be used by ordinary college students or by military personnel to enhance cognitive performance (Chatterjee, 2006; Kadison, 2005; Vastag, 2004), thus raising questions about the validity of AD/HD as a disorder.

In addition to gaps in our understanding of basic mechanisms in psychopharmacology, there are also important lacunae in clinical psychopharmacology. The majority of randomized controlled trials of psychotropics to date have been undertaken in Western adult populations, over the short term, and in tertiary settings. Regulatory authorities require only a few positive trials for an agent to be released on the market, typically for a single indication (such as major depression). There are comparatively few data on the use of psychotropics in other kinds of populations (e.g. children), over the long term, and in general psychiatric or primary settings (Klein *et al.*, 2002; Wells, 1999). For many psychiatric disorders, should a first-line medication fail, there is surprisingly little evidence on which to base the choice of a second-line medication (Fawcett *et al.*, 1999; Stein *et al.*, 2005).

Thus, while the advent of modern psychopharmacology has been a remarkable development, this is a young field, and much additional empirical basic and clinical research remains to be done (Klein, 1993; Klein *et al.*, 2002). Of particular relevance to the current volume is the gap in empirical research on "off-label" indications for psychotropic medications. Once a psychotropic medication is made available, additional data on safety may become available on the basis of post-marketing surveillance. However, the prescription of psychotropics for non-registered conditions (for example, the prescription of an antidepressant for depression that does not meet criteria for a major depression) may continue on the basis of clinical judgement rather than empirical trials. The lack of data in this area contributes to the difficulty of the philosophical questions raised by modern psychopharmacology, the focus of the next chapter.

2

Philosophical questions raised by psychopharmacology

In addition to the many empirical questions that remain for psychopharmacology, the field has raised important philosophical issues for the cognitive and clinical sciences. Philosophy of medicine, philosophy of psychology, and philosophy of cognitive science have only recently begun to address conceptual issues in neuroscience (Bechtel *et al.*, 2001; Bennett & Hacker, 2003; Bickle, 2003; Churchland, 2002; Mishara, 2007), and by and large have ignored the area of clinical psychopharmacology. This volume attempts to begin to address this notable gap in the literature.

A host of philosophical questions are raised by modern psychopharmacology. For the purposes of this volume, these can be divided into (1) conceptual or metaphysical questions about categories relevant to psychopharmacology, (2) explanatory or epistemological questions addressing our knowledge of how psychotropics work, and (3) moral or ethical questions about when psychotropics should be used. In the rest of this chapter I will very briefly outline each of these categories of questions; the rest of the volume will then consider each of these categories and questions in turn, exploring them in more detail.

Conceptual questions raised by the effects of psychotropics

Psychopharmacology raises questions about a number of categories employed in psychiatry. Most importantly, it raises the question of how optimally to define medical and psychiatric disorders.[1] The definition of disorder lies at the heart of philosophy of medicine, and how we think about disorder may well impact on how we think about interventions, including treatment with pharmaceuticals or psychotropics. Some may go so far as to argue that if a particular medical or psychiatric intervention is useful, then this helps define the existence of an underlying medical or psychiatric disorder (Kessler *et al.*, 2003; Reznek, 1988). Is disorder the kind of thing that can be defined in terms of necessary and sufficient conditions (e.g. a *square* has certain essential features), or is it more of a category that mainly reflects particular social practices (e.g. what counts as a *weed* may vary from time to time and place to place)?

A second set of conceptual questions relates to psychotropic medications themselves. The question of how to define a pharmaceutical and a psychotropic are not entirely straightforward. For example, what is the distinction between the use of psychiatric medications for therapy versus enhancement? What are the boundaries between psychiatric medications, legal drugs (alcohol, nicotine), and illicit substances of abuse (cocaine, heroin)? Are nutrients such as the amino acid, tryptophan, which may act to increase serotonergic neurotransmission, best conceptualized as pharmaceuticals (that is, so-called neutraceuticals)? How important is it to draw a distinction between psychotropics that are identical to endogenous compounds and those that act to perturb endogenous mechanisms?

A third set of conceptual questions raised by psychopharmacology is concerned with defining emotions and the self, the person, and his or her character. It seems unproblematic to assert that if an individual imbibes alcohol and acts impulsively or rashly, then a sympathetic audience might characterize this behaviour as out of character. What happens when an individual experiences gradual positive psychological changes in response to a psychotropic, so that they later come to see themselves as having previously suffered from a chronic disorder – have they lived their life "out of character"? These questions in turn raise questions about how best to understand how psychotropics work.

---

[1] I use the term "disorder" rather than "disease" only by convention. The term "disease" connotes an understanding of precise pathology, which is often absent in psychiatric conditions.

Explanatory questions about how psychotropics work

Psychopharmacology raises the epistemological question of how to understand the mind-body in general and psychotropics in particular. Psychopharmacologists have produced a range of neuroscientific data about how psychotropics act to affect one or other biological system (e.g. benzodiazepines act on the γ-aminobutyric acid or GABA receptor). However, it is unclear whether such work fully addresses the question of how these agents work to change thoughts, feelings, and behaviours (how does a benzodiazepine result in reduced anxiety?). Our accounts of how psychotropics work and of how psychotherapy works seem to operate on entirely different levels of discourse (e.g. we describe a psychotropic as altering a neuronal receptor in the brain, but we describe a psychotherapeutic intervention as leading to a change in the patient's way of thinking or feeling). What is the relationship between such views? An immediate possibility is that psychotherapy affects the software of the mind, but that medication affects the hardware – is such a view valid? The problem of understanding how treatment works also raises the related question of understanding how disorders arise, of conceptualizing how genetic and environmental factors underlie pathology.

A second set of explanatory questions relates to placebo and nocebo effects. Clinical psychopharmacology relies on the use of double-blind placebo-controlled trials in which participants are randomized to receive either active medication or an inert substance, with both physician and patient kept "blind" about the identity of the tablet. In such controlled trials, there is often a sizeable clinical response in patients given the inert substance (the placebo effect). Conversely, a remarkable number of subjects experience adverse events in response to administration of an inert substance (the nocebo effect). How should these phenomena best be conceptualized? How should the unconscious processes at play here be characterized?

A final group of explanatory questions about psychotropics involves the discipline of evolutionary psychology. There is a growing literature which argues that thoughts, feelings and behaviours should not merely be explained in terms of their underlying proximal mechanisms, but that it is also relevant to consider their more distal, evolutionary origins

(Cosmides & Tooby, 2003; Laland & Brown, 2002). Increasingly, evolutionary explanations have been applied to medicine in general (Nesse & Williams, 1994) and to psychiatry in particular (Baron-Cohen, 1997; McGuire & Troisi, 1998; Stevens & Price, 1996). Instead of focusing on the proximal factors that underlie pathology, an evolutionary perspective focuses on the distal or evolutionary mechanisms that create vulnerability to disease. Is such a perspective valuable in understanding the effects of psychotropics?

Moral questions about when to use psychotropics

It seems clear that if a patient has a life-threatening pneumonia then it is a reasonable medical decision to administer an effective antibiotic. By analogy, if a person has a life-threatening depression, it seems logical that it is valuable to arrange for a physician to prescribe an effective antidepressant. However, it is unclear whether this argument would hold for a range of other psychiatric symptoms, such as chronic low-grade depressive symptoms (dysthymia), variations in temperament (such as shyness) or behaviours that seem bad rather than mad (for example, impulsive-aggression).

This problem is made particularly acute by the argument that psychological phenomena, including psychiatric symptoms, can be understood as meaningful within their particular phylogenetic and ontogenetic framework (Bolton & Hill, 1996). Apparently negative or destructive emotions, such as shyness, aggression, or jealousy, have important positive features (Goldie, 2000). Similarly, in the realm of cognition there is the phenomenon of depressive realism – people with depression may be more accurate in judging contingencies between responses and outcomes in the world than people without depression (Haaga & Beck, 1995). Pharmacotherapy of cognitive-affective symptoms, perhaps particularly if unaccompanied by the insight that psychotherapy can bring, therefore arguably runs the risk of being harmful.

What about so-called "cosmetic psychopharmacology"? This term was coined by the psychiatrist Peter Kramer, who addressed this potentially new use of psychotropics in his volume *Listening to Prozac*, perhaps the first extended meditation on the conceptual implications of modern psychopharmacology for society and for psychiatry (Kramer, 1997). Pharmaceuticals are used increasingly to enhance athletic or sexual performance (Flower, 2004), and plastic surgery is widely used to enhance physical appearance (Bolt *et al.*, 2002). Is there a rationale for using psychotropics to optimize psychological well-being and function, even in the absence of disorder? If novel agents act to improve memory, decrease shyness, or reduce impulsivity, for example, what are the pros and cons of widespread prescription of such agents?

Considerations about when and how it is appropriate to treat disorders and symptoms cross the fact–value divide (Canguilhem, 1966; de Beaufort *et al.*, 2000; Fulford, 1989; Fulford *et al.*, 2005; Hare, 1983; Pellegrino & Thomasma, 1981; Sadler, 1997, 2002; Schaffner, 1999; Wakefield, 1992b). Furthermore, there is a tension in Western society between values of self-improvement, which would encourage people to use novel technologies including psychotropics, and values around tradition and nature, which argue that such changes are not authentic (Elliott, 2003; Parens, 1998b, 2005). Such debate is stirred by technical breakthroughs such as gene therapy (Anderson, 1989; Jonas, 1974; McGee, 1997; Walters & Palmer, 1997), or the development of selective serotonin reuptake inhibitors such as fluoxetine (Prozac). However, the debate has occurred many times in the past; early psychotropics such as barbiturates,[2] cocaine, and benzodiazepines were initially viewed as having significant value as cosmetic psychotropics that were useful even in those who did not suffer from disorders (Elliott, 2003).

Conclusion

There are a number of philosophical questions that relate to psychopharmacology, but that will not be addressed here, as they arguably involve broader issues in philosophy of medicine and psychiatry, or in philosophy of mind, rather than issues more specifically tied to the philosophy of psychopharmacology per se. These include questions such

---

[2] Barbiturates were perhaps the first synthetic psychotropics marketed as enhancers. In 1863 Adolf van Baeyer synthesized barbituric acid, which he named after his girlfriend Barbara.

as consent with regard to psychotropic medication in research and in the clinic, the use of psychotropic medication to compel truthfulness under interrogation or to end life during euthanasia, and the ethics of animal and stem cell research on psychopharmacology.

On the other hand, the questions raised here will ultimately lead to a whole range of more general philosophical and clinical questions, including questions about how to conceptualize science, language, and mind, about disease and illness, pharmacotherapy and psychotherapy, and placebos and the unconscious. These questions are not the primary focus of the volume, but we need to address them in order to provide a framework for considering the questions raised by psychopharmacology.

While a great deal of work has been done on the philosophy of science, language, mind, and medicine, the intersection between philosophy and psychiatry per se is a more circumscribed one. Relatively little philosophical work has been done in the area of psychopharmacology in general, and cosmetic psychopharmacology in particular.[3] I hope that this volume begins to break some new ground in this area, and by so doing contributes to providing a conceptual foundation for good clinical psychopharmacology.

---

[3] A number of the questions raised by psychopharmacology are also raised by other branches of science in general (e.g. genetics) and neuroscience in particular (e.g. brain imaging). For example, progress in genetics has raised the question of what it means to be 98% chimpanzee (Marks, 2002), and advances in neuro-imaging raise a number of conceptual questions (Fusar-Poli & Broome, 2006). I will refer at times to this parallel literature.

3

How to think about science, language, and medicine: classical, critical, and integrated perspectives

To address specific conceptual questions about psychopharmacology, we first need to consider a number of larger questions about science, about language, about medicine, and even about philosophy. In many ways, this volume is about all of these issues. However, we need to begin with a single starting point, and so we will begin with what is perhaps the most important question in philosophy of medicine: "What is a medical disorder?", and perhaps the most important question in philosophy of psychiatry: "What is a psychiatric disorder?" (Engelhardt, 2000; Engelhardt & Spicker, 1977; Stempsey, 2004).

These turn out to be useful questions-with-which-to-think (Papert, 1980). Beginning with these two questions provides an opportunity to demonstrate the approach taken throughout this volume. First, the two questions are central to medicine and to psychiatry, and so provide a segue into many other issues. Second, there have been well-delineated formal definitions of disorder (the classical approach) as well as a range of arguments that no scientific response is possible (the critical approach); providing a foundation on which a contrasting position can be built here.

The position here draws on cognitive-affective science and emphasizes that the brain-mind is embodied. Over the course of this chapter we will gradually try to reach a conclusion that sensorimotor-affective neuronal circuitry allows humans to interact with their physical and social world, and this in turn leads to the development of basic-level and abstract cognitive-affective maps (or metaphors) for understanding the world. Before we get there, however, in order to clarify the way in which this position contrasts with the classical and critical positions, we need to begin by delineating those positions in more detail. Any attempt to include a whole range of thinkers under a simple rubric must fail, and the aim here is to attempt to show some important family resemblances, rather than to stake out necessary and sufficient criteria for belonging to these divergent schools of thought.

Many prior authors have contrasted two broad schools and so helped shape the argument here (Berlin, 1980; Bhaskar, 1978; Cilliers, 1998; Flanagan, 2003; Keat & Urry, 1982; Suppe, 1974; von Wright, 1971). A series of useful distinctions have been drawn between *erklären* (explanation) and *verstehen* (understanding) (Dilthey, 1883; Jaspers, 1963; Strasser, 1985; van Niekerk, 1989; von Wright, 1971), tough-minded and tender-minded (James, 1907), objectivism and intellectualism (Merleau-Ponty, 1942), platonism and nominalism (Quine, 1969), metaphysicists and ironists (Rorty, 1979), objectivism and relativism (Bernstein, 1983; Harman & Thomson, 1996; Johnson, 1993),[1] rationalism and romanticism (Gellner, 1985), universalism and historicism (Margolis, 1986), positivism and antirealism (Miller, 1987), the nomological and the idiographic (Schwartz & Wiggins, 1987), the modern and the post-modern (Bertens, 1995), empiricism and post-empiricism (Bolton & Hill, 1996), essentialism and normativism (Schaffner, 1999), and the objective and the reactive (Elliott, 2003). The differentiation here will begin by focusing on the different approaches of the classical and critical schools to categories in general, and then on their different approaches to the category of disorder in particular. In later parts of the volume, we will also focus in greater detail on differences in their approach to explanation, and to ethics.

---

[1] Johnson (1993) mostly refers to absolutism rather than objectivism. One summary of this broad range of contrasts, listed here according to year of publication, would be in terms of their accounts of (general and medical) entities (objective vs. subjective, essentialism vs. nominalism), accounts (explanation vs. understanding, disease vs. illness) and values (absolutism vs. relativism, medicine as science vs. humanity).

Classical and critical approaches – algorithms vs. narratives

Madness need not be regarded as an illness. Why shouldn't it be seen as a sudden – more or less sudden – change of character. (Wittgenstein)

Abigail Adams one day saw a newspaper advertisement aimed at people who worry about embarrassing themselves when they have to talk in front of others, or go to small gatherings and parties. She had felt uncomfortable in social situations for as long as she could remember and read further with interest. The advert had been placed by researchers at a local medical school, and she decided to make an appointment to learn more. At the appointment she met Dr Bapela Bamanzini, who told Abigail that she suffered from a condition called social anxiety disorder. On her way home, Abigail was somewhat sceptical; she had always known that she was reserved, but she felt that in many ways this trait was a valuable asset.

A classical approach to categorization holds that membership in categories can be described in terms of necessary and sufficient characteristics (Smith & Medin, 1981). For example, a square is defined as having four features: (1) four sides; (2) four angles; (3) all sides are equal; and (4) all angles are equal; all members of this category are homogeneous insofar as each has all of these defining attributes. Furthermore, the category of squares exists independently of people, and independently of the characteristics of human categorizers.

This kind of approach to science and to language has roots in Plato's work, was adopted by logical positivism and the early Wittgenstein, and continues to be enormously influential in Anglo-American analytic philosophy (Lakoff & Johnson, 1999; Varela *et al.*, 1991). This approach has also strongly influenced particular schools in psychology and psychiatry; in particular, behaviourism, certain schools of psychoanalysis, and symbolic cognitivism. Although thinkers within this tradition differ markedly from one another, common themes are that science is comprised of formal laws, that language entails the use of specifiable terms, and that mind involves the processing of symbols.

The idea that science is comprised of formal laws has a long history. Plato (427–347 BC) held that knowledge was best exemplified by mathematics, and that understanding reality involved a priori reasoning to discover the abstract objects that existed in a timeless "realm of the intellect" ("Plato's Heaven"). Mill, in a particularly important work of nineteenth-century positivism, emphasized the uniformity of the laws of nature, arguing that the scientific method comprises inducing laws from empirical data (Mill, 1843).[2] Frege and Russell, at the turn of the twentieth century, attempted to reduce mathematics to logic, arguing that logic is a complex structure resting on a finite set of basic elements, and that rules or algorithms could then be used to produce more complex structures.

A classical approach has often held that the universal method of science includes the study of both physical and human phenomena, including those related to health and illness. Mill (1843), for example, argued that scientific laws applied equally to physical and psychological events. This position often includes a reductionistic element, which argues that the most basic and important laws are those formulated in the physical sciences (Neurath *et al.*, 1969). In this perspective, physical and psychological phenomena can be studied in the same scientific way, and a definition of medical disorders and of psychiatric disorders can follow essentially the same form. This approach was taken by early authors in the philosophy of medicine and psychiatry (Boorse, 1976a; Hempel, 1965), and it continues to be followed by influential thinkers (Wakefield, 1992a).

A classical approach to language holds that meaning can be fully specified in terms of our direct knowledge of the world, and subsequent definitions and logic. Hume distinguished between "matters of fact" and "relations of ideas" (Hume, 1739), while Kant contrasted synthetic and analytic judgements (Kant, 1781); laying the foundation for the idea that the sentences which comprise human knowledge are true by virtue of the facts of the world, or true by virtue of the meanings of their terms. Carnap and other logical positivists went on to argue that

---

[2] Bacon and the English empiricists (Locke, Berkeley, Hume) influenced Comte, who in turn influenced Mill's view of the continuity between the methods of the natural and human sciences. Mill's book can be considered as having set off the *methodenstreit* in Germany. I later also briefly discuss the implications of a "unified conception of science" for biology.

analysis of the meaning of terms is key not only for understanding logic, but also for addressing broader philosophical questions. Ayer, working in the linguistic-analytic tradition, not only attempted to put forward a principle of verification (an empirical statement is not meaningful unless some empirical observation is relevant to its truth or falsity), but also argued that philosophy is an activity of analysis (of words and their meanings) and so identical with the logic of science (Ayer, 1936).[3]

Classical approaches to science and language have influenced several views in philosophy of mind and in clinical psychology. An early view in philosophy of mind was that mental and physical concepts belong to different categories, but mental states can be analysed in terms of dispositions to behave (Ryle, 1949).[4] A more recent position conceptualizes the mind in terms of the processing of symbols; the mind is functionally analogous to the rules (software) running on a computer (hardware) (Fodor, 1975; Putnam, 1967). In psychology, behaviourists have argued that psychological science should focus on determining the laws that describe the relationship between stimuli and responses. Some psychoanalysts have emphasized the importance of describing unconscious rules that produce human thoughts, feelings and behaviours. Symbolic cognitivists have argued that the mind can be understood as a system of internal representations (Fodor, 1987). Despite the important differences between these psychological schools, their proponents emphasize the rules and algorithms which govern behaviours and representations.

One of the earliest attempts to define the category of medical disorder from a classical approach was that of Boorse (1975, 1976a, 1997), who argued that medical disorders can be defined in terms of malfunction. Working in the same tradition, a range of authors have attempted to further refine this definition (Caplan et al., 1981; Carson & Burns, 1997; Humber & Almeder, 1997; Sadler et al., 1994) and to employ it in the clinic (American Psychiatric Association, 1994; Kendell, 1975; Klein, 1978; Spitzer & Endicott, 1978), and in health planning (Daniels, 1994; Sabin & Daniels, 1994). Although the classical view has predominantly argued for a view of medical disorders as value-free, Wakefield

---

[3] Ayer's volume was important in introducing logical positivism to the English-speaking world.
[4] Ryle's logical behaviourism was influenced by the work of psychological behaviourists.

has suggested that while "dysfunction" can be defined in a value-free way, the concept of disorder necessarily entails a negative evaluation, so that medical disorders can be defined in terms of "harmful dysfunction" (Wakefield, 1992a). Subsequently he has argued strenuously and elegantly that this formal definition covers the necessary and sufficient characteristics of disorder (Wakefield, 1993, 1995, 1997, 1999a, 1999b, 2001). There are close links between a classical view of disorder, and the "medical model" (Macklin, 1973), which focuses on physical causes of disorder, and on technical interventions.

A more critical approach argues that categorization is a social practice, and that categories reflect ways of life, indicative of human interests, rather than universal forms. Certainly, we should be aware of the "fallacy of misplaced concreteness", which warns us not to reify abstract categories of thought (Whitehead, 1948). A critical approach is central to a strand of philosophy that stands in opposition to traditional thought, but that also has long historical roots, was re-invigorated by the later Wittgenstein, became central to continental and post-modernist philosophy, and continues to comprise a crucial strand of contemporary thought about science and language, particularly in continental philosophy and in post-modern movements (Bhaskar, 1979; Bolton & Hill, 1996).

This approach has also strongly influenced particular schools in psychology and psychiatry, including phenomenology, interpersonal schools of psychoanalysis, and situated cognitivism. Although thinkers within this tradition differ markedly from one another, common themes are that all observation is theory-laden (what scientists observe necessarily reflects their pre-existing views), that knowledge of humans requires a subjective understanding (scientists are necessarily participants in the human interactions that they observe, rather than simply objective outsiders), that language reflects its speakers' way of life so that meaning cannot be reduced to formal rules, and that the mind can only be understood in terms of the context and culture of the individual to whom it belongs.

Vico and Herder were key figures in the critical tradition, laying the ground for the emphasis on understanding (*verstehen*) in the knowledge of humans (rather than merely explanation (*erklären*)). A focus on

narratives and their interpretation has continued to play an important role in a critical approach in the philosophy of science. A critical
approach to the philosophy of science argues that science itself comprises merely one way of reading the world, and is a perspective that is
not necessarily more privileged than any other. Thus "scientists (even
physical scientists) are a fickle lot", and the history of science "is a tale
of multifarious shiftings of allegiance from theory to theory" (Feyerabend, 1975), as its paradigms (Kuhn, 1971) and programmes (Lakatos,
1978) change over the course of time, partly in accordance with shifts
in power (Barnes, 1974; Bloor, 1991; Bourdieu, 1998; Collins, 1985;
Latour & Woolgar, 1992; Longino, 1990).

A critical approach to language argues that language reflects a
speaker's way of life, and meaning cannot be reduced to formal rules.
Particular statements reflect not only observations, but also a range
of theoretical assumptions (Quine, 1960). Furthermore, insofar as
speakers are situated in the world and speech is intentional, sentences
comprise more than mere representations. In Searle's Chinese room
experiment, for example, he notes that even if a computer is expert
at manipulating Chinese and English symbols, translating the one language to the other, it is nevertheless unable to understand either (Searle,
1983). A continental tradition puts a great deal of emphasis on language,
not with the aim of discovering logical truths, but rather because of its
emphasis on the narratives (including scientific texts) and discursive
practices which shape societies and individuals. This emphasis shifts
the logic of verification to a logic of validation (van Niekerk, 1989).

Critical approaches to science and language have influenced several
views in philosophy of mind and in psychology. Philosophers have
emphasized that by focusing only on observable stimuli and responses,
behaviourism ignores the crucial realm of human subjective experience (Strawson, 1974; van Niekerk, 1986). Furthermore, a range of
thinkers including Wittgenstein (1967), have argued that purely repre-
sentational accounts fail to account for the intentionality (Brentano,
1973) of mental states (Davidson, 1984; Dennett, 1987; McDowell,
1998). A discursive turn in psychology has emphasized that psychological phenomena cannot be reduced to brain events or computational
states, but instead are crucially dependent on interpersonal processes

(Harré & Gillett, 1994). Some psychoanalytic theoretists have conceptualized psychotherapy in terms of narrative text, have emphasized the
intersubjective aspects of analytic phenomena such as the transference,
or have focused on the discursive nature of the unconscious (Habermas,
1971; Klein, 1976; Mitchell, 1988; Ricoeur, 1970, 1981; Schafer, 1976).
Situated cognitivists have emphasized that cognition occurs within a
particular context (Gibson, 1977; Neisser, 1976), and have focused on
computational models, such as neural networks or robotic agents that
operate within particular environments, which allow cognition to be
embodied, and which blur the software–hardware distinction (Clark,
1997; Dreyfus, 2005; Ramsay *et al.*, 1991). Despite important differences between psychological schools that take a critical position, they
emphasise that psychological phenomena cannot be specified in terms
of rules and algorithms, but rather involve multilayered narratives and
discursive practices (Bennett & Hacker, 2003; Harré & Gillett, 1994).

Similarly, many authors have emphasized that medical disorders are
social constructs.[5] They argue that categorizing any particular phenomenon as a disorder reflects cultural and historical theories and values, rather than any underlying universal truth about the relevant phenomenon. This kind of approach has arguably been particularly useful
in studies of medical history and medical anthropology; the hindsight
provided by history and the farsightedness provided by anthropology
throw the theory-bound and value-bound aspects of medicine, including psychopharmacotherapy, into sharp relief.[6] Lilienfeld and Marino
(1995, 1999) provide perhaps the most comprehensive philosophical
response to Wakefield's essentialist analysis (and certainly the one which

---

[5] Ironically, Virchow, a pathologist who made significant contributions to understanding the
cellular basis of disease, was one of the first to recognize this. Thus he wrote, "What we call
disease is solely an abstract concept with the help of which we separate particular
phenomena of daily life from all others, without there being a separation in nature itself".
Similarly, he argued, "Medicine is a social science, and politics nothing but medicine on a
large scale" (quoted in Porter (1997)).

[6] A range of authors have contributed to this literature (Canguilhem, 1966; Conrad &
Schneider, 1980; Davis, 1995b; Doyal, 1979; Ehrenreich & English, 1973; Farmer, 2003;
Foucault, 1973; Holmes *et al.*, 2006; Illich, 1977; Kutchins & Kirk, 1997; Packard, 1977;
Parsons, 1951; Rothman, 1997; Schaler, 2004; Showalter, 1987; Sontag, 1977; Staiano, 1979;
Szasz, 1972; Zola, 1972).

he regards as the most important alternative (Wakefield, 1999a)). They argue that the category of disorder is based on socially constructed prototypes rather than universal natural kinds, and conclude that there is no scientific way of deciding what does and what does not fall in this category. There are close links between critiques of the classical view of disorder, and the attempt to replace the pathology-centred "medical model" with an emphasis on detailing the experience of illness, understanding its emergence within a meaningful context, and providing more comprehensive and holistic approaches to intervention, including an emphasis on the doctor–patient relationship and on social change (Gadamer, 1993; Greenhalgh & Hurwitz, 1998; Kriel, 2000; Leder, 1984; Tauber, 2006; van Leeuwen & Kimsma, 1997).[7]

The question, "what is a medical disorder?", raises the parallel question, "what is a psychiatric disorder?", and the orthogonal question of whether medical and psychiatric disorders should be defined in the same way. This in turn raises the more fundamental questions of naturalism; should the human "sciences" be conceptualized in the same way as the natural sciences, and should they proceed in the same way? These questions in turn lie at the heart of the philosophy of the social sciences in general (Bhaskar, 1979; Harré, 1986a; Keat & Urry, 1982; Piaget, 1970; Sayer, 2000) and of philosophy of psychiatry in particular (Bolton & Hill, 1996; Hundert, 1989; Jaspers, 1963).

A classical approach has held that the categories of science can be conceptualized in terms of a universal theory and method that includes the study of both physical and human phenomena. In this perspective, physical and psychological phenomena can be studied in the same scientific way, and a definition of medical disorders and of psychiatric disorders can follow essentially the same form. As noted earlier, this approach was taken by early authors in the philosophy of medicine and psychiatry (Boorse, 1976a; Hempel, 1965), and it continues to be followed by influential thinkers (Wakefield, 1992a). Hempel, for example, challenged nosologists to provide a classification that carves nature at its joints, and to use operational criteria (Bridgman, 1927).

---

[7] Although the medical model is often referred to as Cartesian, debate about whether behavioural disturbance is best understood as "medical" or "moral" goes back at least to Plato (Kenny, 1969; Simon, 1978).

A classical approach to psychology, combined with a classical approach to somatic and psychological disorder, underpins a number of models in clinical psychiatry, particularly the so-called organic model. In this model, psychiatric disorders are viewed as essentialist entities, caused by internal dysfunction, objectively diagnosable, and deserving of individual treatment (Macklin, 1973; Zachar & Kendler, 2007). This model has its origins in the success of the germ theory of disease, and argues that specific lesions in brain regions or systems lead to psychopathology. Proponents of the organic model emphasize the links between psychiatry and neurology, often referring to psychiatric disorders as brain disorders (Guze, 1989).

A more critical approach, however, has argued against the idea that social studies, including psychiatry, are best understood as sciences. Several authors have argued that both medicine and psychiatry reflect social practices, so that concepts of psychiatric disorder are theory-bound and value-laden (Engelhardt, 2000; Fulford, 1989; Gillett, 1999; Kovacs, 1998; Lilienfeld & Marino, 1995; Margolis, 1976; Nordenfelt, 1995; Reznek, 1988; Sadler, 2002; Toulmin, 1997). Some proponents of a critical position accept the argument that medical disorders can be defined in universal terms, but argue against naturalism, noting that psychiatric classification cuts nature at joints that merely reflect human practices and interests, and so conclude that psychiatric disorders involve a category fallacy, with the metaphors of medicine incorrectly extended to cover psychological phenomena (Ingleby, 1981; Sedgwick, 1982).

A critical approach to psychology, combined with a critical approach to psychological disorders, underpins a number of models in psychiatric practice, particularly those that emphasize patients' narratives and experiences. In such clinical models, a narrow focus on psychiatric disorder is considered reductionistic; instead, the emphasis is on understanding patients as agents who develop meaningful symptoms, within the context of their particular histories and environments (Harré & Gillett, 1994; Zachar & Kendler, 2007). A merger between psychiatry and neurology is therefore far from simple (Pies, 2006). Such views may also downplay the contemporary emphasis on evidence-based medicine and evidence-based psychiatry as overly simplistic or wholly flawed, and emphasize instead the importance of the service user movements and the value of a self-help culture (Bracken, 2003; Bracken & Thomas, 2005; Lewis, 2006).

In summary, the question of whether or not Abigail has a disorder leads to two important traditions of thought which provide contrasting approaches to the general question "what is category x?", and to the more specific questions, "what is a medical disorder?" and "what is a psychiatric disorder?" A classical tradition, often exemplified in Anglo-American analytic philosophy, emphasizes the algorithms and rules underlying science, language, and the mind, and attempts to define rigorously the necessary and sufficient characteristics of categories such as disorder, explaining them according to formal rules, and holding that they are value-free. A critical tradition, on the other hand, often exemplified by philosophers influenced by the later Wittgenstein, continental philosophy, and anti-psychiatry theory, emphasizes the contextuality and subjectivity inherent in science, language and the mind, explaining them in terms of multilayered narratives, and holding that our concepts and explanations are bound up with our values.

A naturalist approach – Roschian categories and the embodied brain-mind

In discussing the question of how we know whether someone who is holding his cheek has toothache, Wittgenstein writes, ". . . what if we went on asking: – 'And why do you suppose that toothache corresponds to his holding his cheek just because your toothache corresponds to your holding your cheek?' You will be at a loss to answer this question, and find that here we strike rock bottom, that is we have come down to conventions." What exactly does Wittgenstein mean by 'conventions' here? When we have toothache, we find that certain responses tend to follow – for example, crying out, holding our cheeks, etc. By convention, the word "pain" is taken to describe this set of responses – "pain" is what makes us cry out, hold our cheeks, etc. (Harrison, 1979)[8]

---

[8] Wittgenstein's discussion here is in the *Blue Book*, pp. 24–6 (Wittgenstein, 1960), although he also addresses pain in *Philosophical Investigations* (Wittgenstein, 1967). Harrison holds that Wittgenstein is not making a behaviourist argument, nor solely emphasizing that language involves conventions, but rather is arguing for a continuity between the conventions of language and the nature of the world.

The classical approach may be criticized for failing to recognize that science and medicine are social practices, and that definitions of disorder are necessarily theory-bound and value-laden. Conversely, the critical approach may be criticized for failing to recognize that science and medicine are not entirely subjective or relativistic, but that the theories and values reflected in medical and psychiatric nomenclatures can be rationally debated. On the basis of this kind of philosophical reasoning, a number of authors have argued for an approach which acknowledges that natural and social sciences are social practices, but also allows that natural and social sciences provide knowledge of real structures and their mechanisms (Bhaskar, 1978) and functions (Bolton & Hill, 1996). Such an approach attempts to avoid both the charges of "scientism" and "cynicism" (Haack, 2003).

While natural science may provide an understanding of kinds that reflect the essence of nature's structures and mechanisms, social science cuts nature at joints that instead reflect human practices and interests, and the emergent phenomena of more complex sciences cannot be fully specified in the terms of more basic sciences (Bhaskar, 1979). Complex brain-mind phenomena, such as pain, need to be investigated with a range of theories and methods (Degenaar, 1979; Jaspers, 1963; Panksepp, 1998). Such an approach to natural and human science arguably then forms the basis for an integrative and realist view of the sciences (Bhaskar, 1978), for a non-reductionistic naturalist approach to psychology (Manicas & Secord, 1983), and for a view on categorizing medical and psychiatric disorder that goes beyond the classical and critical perspectives (Stein, 1991).

Are there any data which can be used to support such an apparently attractive and synthetic position? It turns out that a range of empirical data can now inform our view of categories in general and the category of disorder in particular. Cognitive science as initially conceptualized incorporated cognitive psychology, linguistics, artificial intelligence, neuroscience, anthropology, and philosophy (Gardner, 1985), and we will explore next the way in which each of these sub-disciplines has tackled the general question of categorization. In addition, we add developmental psychology, and evolutionary psychology, two increasingly important fields in the cognitive-affective sciences.

Cognitive psychology has emphasized that categories are not homogenous, but rather have central and peripheral exemplars (Rosch, 1978). Prototypes are category members which serve as the most central, or typical exemplars. For example, when presented with a list of different birds (robin, owl, ostrich), research subjects agree fairly consistently on which kinds of birds are typical birds (e.g. robin), which are less typical (e.g. owl), and which are atypical (e.g. ostrich). Typical exemplars, or birds that lie at the centre of the category, may have such attributes as having feathers and wings, and being able to fly and sing; atypical exemplars may not. Different experimental paradigms, including reaction times, production of examples, and similarity ratings, confirm that many categories have graded structures. Categories are intimately related to human actions and activities.

Linguistics has provided additional evidence that abstract categories (such as disorder) are crucially dependent on neuronally based sensorimotor and affective experience (such as the experience of pain). Lakoff's elegant analyses point to the existence of what he terms radial categories, made up of a central case (based on basic-level sensorimotor–affective experience) and conventionalized variations (requiring metaphoric extensions or mappings from the central case; Lakoff, 1987). For example, the central case in the category of mothers describes a female who gives birth to a child, supplies half of the child's genes, nurtures the child, and so on. Variations on the central case include such entities as stepmother, adoptive mother, birth mother, or foster mother, which lack one or more attributes of the central case. In addition, Lakoff emphasizes that complex abstract concepts (such as marriage) are structured in terms of more basic-level metaphors (e.g. MARRIAGE as a JOURNEY). Thus linguistics suggests that the brain-mind relies on prototypes and metaphors grounded in human experience, rather than on the formal manipulation of abstract representations (Piattelli-Palmarini, 1980).

The field of artificial intelligence can potentially provide useful models of categorization. In particular, connectionist models are able to show how simple neural networks process complex graded and radial categories (Churchland, 1995; Ramsay et al., 1991; Rumelhart et al., 1986). Consider, for example, a neural network that classifies faces. It turns out that such a neural network has minima for male and female faces that are based not on necessary and sufficient criteria, but rather on a graded kind of pattern recognition. The parallel distributed processing of such networks is characterized by several features that may be important in simulating categorization: cognitive-affective processing in the absence of central control; processing in parallel rather than serially; content-addressable memory rather than memory located by an abstract name; relatively slow processing in individual units in contrast with rapid processing in the whole network; processing by different areas of interacting modules using reciprocal connections; learning via adjustment of synaptic strengths; efficient pattern recognition; and graceful degeneration rather than sudden crashing of the system after disturbances to the network (Norman, 1986). More recently, sophisticated, biologically based robotic and connectionist models have helped explain how the brain-mind grounds meaning in perception and action, and relies on embodied prototypes rather than solely on binary rule-like representations (O'Reilly, 2006; Roy, 2005).

Work in neuroscience and anthropology can be used to determine the lower- and higher-level constraints on categorization; this is seen, for example, in work on colour classification (Berlin & Kay, 1969; Kay & McDaniel, 1978). Languages do not simply carve up the colour spectrum in arbitrary ways; some languages employ highly differentiated classification of basic colours (up to 11 basic colours), while others have little differentiation (cool vs. warm colours). While the boundaries between colour ranges differ from language to language, focal colours are classified in highly regular ways by speakers of languages with the same colour category differentiation. Thus, in languages with a basic term for the range of blue colours, all speakers choose the same focal blue as the best example of blue. Colour categorization is a product of human neurophysiology and culturally specific cognitive-affective operations; our categories are embodied in neuronal circuits which mediate our sensorimotor-affective experience of the physical and social world.[9]

---

[9] The idea that similar processes underlie the perception of action, action, and social cognition has been termed the "motor theory of social cognition". Such an account may be particularly relevant for basic-level processing (Hurley, 1998; O'Regan & Noë, 2001), although complex cognitive-affective processing may not be reducible to motor processes (Gallagher, 2005).

Evolutionary theory (with its focus on phylogenesis) is increasingly contributing to cognitive-affective science. In general, the idea is that the brain-mind has evolved to optimize the way in which particular organisms make their living (Duchaine *et al.*, 2001; Papineau, 2003; Ruse, 1995). In all animals, the nervous system contributes to homeostasis by approaching rewarding stimuli and avoiding punishing ones. In the case of humans, our brain-minds have specialized in complex decision-making, including planning the future. For such purposes it may be useful to include self-representation (see later chapter on the self). However, at a simpler level, it turns out that humans make finer discriminations between greenish, yellowish, and orangish colours than they do in bluish regions. At a proximal level, this can be explained by the neurophysiology of vision. But at a distal level, there are evolutionary reasons for this human capacity. Other species, which have different ways of living in the world, have different neurophysiologies, and discriminate better amongst different colours than do humans.

Developmental cognitive-affective science (with its focus on onto-genesis) may also contribute to understanding categories. The idea that neuronal circuits involved in sensorimotor-affective experience (e.g. of pain) are used to structure basic and abstract categories (e.g. disorder) has early roots in psychology (Piaget, 1952; Vygotsky, 1934). Connectionist models are able to show how neural networks learn. Such work highlights how the brain-mind can make simple kinds of categorization early on, but over time, with more participation in the world, it can make highly abstract differentiations (Mareschal *et al.*, 2007). Such work shows that categories, like other cognitive-affective phenomena, cannot be understood in terms of simply nature or nurture, but rather reflect a complex interaction between genetic and environmental variables. Colour categorizations reflect the molecular genetics of our visual system, but also particular cultural approaches to colour classification.

What can philosophy contribute to cognitive science? One idea is that philosophy puts forward the ideas first, and cognitive science repeats them (Fodor, 2000). Certainly, thought experiments have long been used to demonstrate that human categories are fuzzy at the edges. The physician-philosopher Locke, for example, distinguished between what he termed nominal and real essences, and argued that there are no fixed boundaries in nature (Locke, 1694). Similary, the notion that the brain-mind is situated in the body and its interaction with the world is an old one. Spinoza, for example, noted that "The Mind does not have the capacity to perceive . . . except in so far as it perceives the ideas of the modifications (affections) of the body" (de Spinoza, 1677).[10] Kant made an attempt to describe schemas as structures that while internal, were modified in response to the experience of the external world, a position that is partially consistent with much modern cognitive-affective science (Kant, 1781).[11]

Similarly, the later Wittgenstein (1967) emphasized that representations do not simply mirror the world, but rather that concepts involve sets of family resemblances, they are tied to our interests, and their meaning is grounded in social activity; a position that has since been drawn upon to argue for the modern cognitivist view that information is encoded in the brain-mind (Bolton & Hill, 1996). Alongside such work, continental philosophy has developed a concept of the lived-body (Merleau-Ponty, 1963b); the body does not merely involve mechanically caused acts; rather, it is an intentional entity that "understands" the world by perceiving its surroundings and moving towards goals. Merleau-Ponty (1962) and Straus (1963), for example, have both emphasized that sensory perception cannot be reduced to the Cartesian alternatives of merely a mechanical process or a disembodied type of thought, but rather involves a bodily intelligence and affectivity, a body-subject, a "being-in-the-world".[12] This kind of thinking has

---

[10] Whereas Descartes's thinking was imbued with physics, Spinoza had a particularly biological perspective. Hampshire argues that this had a number of consequences for Spinoza's unique contributions, including his preference for descriptions of individual natures rather than of universal laws, his notions of physical and psychological explanation (akin to *erklären* vs. *verstehen*), and his view that the vocabulary we use for ethics should be the same that we use for describing nature (Hampshire, 2005).

[11] Kant has a chapter on "schematism" in the *Critique of Pure Reason*. He discusses how there must be some connection between the experienced idea and the experienced world, the schema is "properly, only the phenomenon, or sensible concept, of an object in agreement with the category". Thus despite an attempt to reconcile rationalism and empiricism, his view is rather different from the cognitive-affective science construct of an embodied schema.

[12] "Being-in-the world" can be contrasted with Sartre's "being-in-itself" (or matter) and "being-for-itself" (or mind). Note also Bourdieu's view of *habitus* – the socialized body, or the individual's physiological incorporation of social norms (Bourdieu, 1998).

provided a foundation for the so-called "corporeal turn" in a broad range of contemporary theoretical work which emphasizes the importance of embodiment in social practices (Witz, 2000).

Thus, a range of disciplines within the cognitive-affective sciences, including philosophy, provide increasingly sophisticated ideas and data, on the embodied brain-mind and its categories (Churchland, 2002; Clark, 1997; Gibbs, 2006; Varela *et al.*, 1991; Wheeler, 2005). The current volume rests on the shoulders of authors who have suggested ways of going beyond the classical versus critical divide by understanding how categories or cognitive-affective maps emerge from the interaction of our brain-minds with the physical and social world, by emphasizing the continuity between philosophical work on these kinds of notions of embodiment and subsequent cognitive-affective science data on the centrality of embodiment to brain-mind processes, and by suggesting the possibility of a naturalized philosophy at the intersection of conceptual and empirical work on the brain-mind (Bolton & Hill, 1996; Churchland, 2002; Clark, 1997; Gallagher, 2005; Lakoff & Johnson, 1999; Varela *et al.*, 1991).

With the range of data from cognitive-affective science in mind, we can return to our general question, "what is the category x?", and to our specific question, "what is a disorder?" These data allow one to go beyond the classical and critical approaches, by showing that categories, like other cognitive-affective phenomena, are embodied in the neuronal circuits of the brain-mind, and in its interactions with the world (Bolton & Hill, 1996; Lakoff & Johnson, 1999; Varela *et al.*, 1991). While it may be possible to define some categories in terms of natural kinds that exist independently of humans (Kripke, 1980; Putnam, 1975), many categories are explicitly tied to human practices and interests (Fulford, 1989; Thornton, 2002). Thus, abstract categories like disorder cannot be defined in terms of formal rules that describe necessary and sufficient criteria (as posited in the classical approach), nor can they be viewed as entirely open to interpretation (as argued in the critical approach), but rather should be understood as emerging from sensorimotor-affective experience (e.g. of pain) and resultant cognitive-affective mapping.

For the purposes of this volume, we do not need a very detailed understanding of the mechanisms by which categories emerge and operate, but in the next section the work of Lakoff and Johnson (1999) is drawn on in order to provide a framework for considering how the category of disorder is structured. This approach is then used to consider the range of conceptual problems raised by modern psychopharmacology.

The category of disorder – the data on disorder as metaphor

(A) *Conrad Cleese is a young man living in the twenty-first century. He is in good health; indeed, he eats a balanced diet, exercises regularly, and does not smoke. One morning he wakes up, notes that he has a fever and a cough, and feels too ill to go to work. Conrad calls a doctor who diagnoses a bacterial throat infection, prescribes an antibiotic, and books him off work. After a few days of treatment he is well enough to return to work.*

(B) *David Donaldson is a young man who is a slave on a plantation in the American South in the early nineteenth century. After a series of alter-cations with his master, he gradually begins to demonstrate discipline problems, and is ultimately caught attempting to run away. A doctor is called, a diagnosis of drapetomania is made, and strong discipline and labour are prescribed. David remains under close observation for a long time, for fear his drapetomania will return.*

How is the category of disorders structured – which sensorimotor-affective structures are used to construct relevant basic-level cognitive-affective maps, and how are these then combined and extended to pro-vide abstract understandings of disorder? This question is perhaps best addressed by rigorous empirical studies (Campbell *et al.*, 1979). Nev-ertheless, even a superficial exploration of Western concepts yields a number of pertinent mappings of disorder: disorder as involving war-fare, disorder as contamination, disorder as impediment, disorder as breakdown, and disorder as imbalance. (In other cultures, a range of other mappings, including disorder as ancestral intervention, may also be common.) Each of these metaphors entails a view (or a schema) of cause, effect, and treatment of the disorder. Thus, we have the following:

DISORDER as WARFARE/BATTLE[13]
> Cause: Enemy
> Effect: Defeat
> Treatment: Weapons

DISORDER as CONTAMINATION
> Cause: Pollutant
> Effect: Contamination
> Treatment: Cleansing agent

DISORDER as IMPEDIMENT[14]
> Cause: Blockage
> Effect: Stumbling
> Treatment: Overcoming blockage

DISORDER as BREAKDOWN
> Cause: Breakage
> Effect: Breakdown
> Treatment: Fixing breakdown

DISORDER as IMBALANCE[15]
> Cause: Novel stressor
> Effect: Disruption of homeostasis
> Treatment: Restore balance

A first point to be made here is that the category of disorder has a graded structure, with some exemplars central and others peripheral. Conrad Cleese's infection, presented earlier, represents a central, prototypical exemplar of medical disorder. The centrality of this case is enhanced by the ready identification of an external cause, which in turn results

---

[13] Both the DISORDER as WARFARE/BATTLE and the DISORDER as CONTAMINATION metaphors can be conceptualized as variants of the OBJECT (possession) version of the more general EVENT STRUCTURE metaphor (Lakoff & Johnson, 1999).

[14] Both the DISORDER as IMPEDIMENT and the DISORDER as BREAKDOWN metaphors can be conceptualized as variants of the LOCATION (pathway) version of the more general EVENT STRUCTURE metaphor (Lakoff & Johnson, 1999).

[15] Imbalance is what Johnson terms an image schema (Johnson, 1993). Metaphors of IMBALANCE and JOURNEY are often combined to explain a psychological struggle (Johnson, 1993).

in negative somatic effects, for which standard medical interventions are available. Thus the mapping or metaphors of disorder seem to fit Conrad's infection well (perhaps because infection is a phenomenon to which our sensorimotor-affective apparatus is so acutely attuned). The warfare metaphor, for example, clearly applies: there is an enemy (bacterium) that attacks the body, resulting in a breach of the body's (immunological) defences, until additional reinforcements from the (medical) armamentarium are brought to bear.[16]

Lay people would readily agree that Conrad is suffering from a medical disorder, and invoke related social practices (seminally defined in terms of the "sick role"). The fact that his disorder is due to an external force that is transformative, that he had no personal responsibility for it, and that standard medical interventions exist, all contribute to the acceptability of categorizing his infection as a disorder, rather than as some other kind of deviance (Parsons, 1951). Similarly, classical philosophers are likely to view Conrad as suffering from a disorder; Boorse's definition of medical disorder as a malfunction, for example, turns out to be very similar to the commonly used mapping of this category as a breakdown (Boorse, 1975). Such similarities between philosophical constructs and lay mappings strengthen the acceptability of conceptual analysis, and make it harder to point out the ways in which its metaphors are not always apt (Lakoff & Johnson, 1999).

A range of disorders are, however, more peripheral, and more atypical than Conrad's bacterial throat infection. These include disorders where there is no external transformative factor (so that the deviance seems merely a normal variation), where the person may have some responsibility for what has happened (e.g. obesity, alcoholism), and where interventions other than medical ones are standard (e.g. spiritual interventions for ageing, legal interventions for psychopathy). In the case of David Donaldson, for example, it is difficult to apply the mappings of disorder; there is no apparent enemy or pollutant to account for his behaviour. Instead mappings and metaphors that revolve around escape and freedom are clearly more pertinent.

---

[16] Psychological trauma plays a crucial role in the typical case of mental disorder; this is seen, for example, in the early work of both Freud and Watson.

Lay people, too, would be loath to accept that David has a disorder, or to invoke the sick role. His desire to escape would seem to be part of who he is (rather than the result of a transformative force), among friends he would own responsibility for his acting on this wish, and there is no standard medical intervention for wanting freedom; these points all make it difficult to categorize his behaviour as a disorder, and make it easier to see it as (heroically) breaking the law of the time. Similarly, the argument of critical philosophers that the label of "drapetomania" says more about the theories and values of Southern slave owners than about David's bid for freedom (Cartwright, 1981; Kutchins & Kirk, 1997) seems entirely valid. Despite critical philosophers' attempt to deconstruct the category of disorders, it turns out that there is surprising overlap between philosophical constructs and lay mappings (this time of non-disorders).

In the realist and embodied approach taken in this volume, the category of disorder should not be understood in terms of a classical kind with necessary and sufficient characteristics, but rather can be depicted in terms of particular cognitive-affective mappings which reflect our interaction with the physical and social world. The view of metaphor taken here is quite different from those which focus on the observable features of physical and mental disorder (Pickering, 2006; Szasz, 1972); it emphasizes that our abstract constructs and their meanings are embedded in and enacted by the brain-mind. The more prototypic the illness (i.e. the more closely the exemplar, such as Conrad's infection or posttraumatic stress disorder, is covered by the standard metaphors of disease outlined above), the more unconscious are our mappings, and the more difficult it is to see the relevant theories and values at hand. The less prototypic the illness (i.e. the more these standard metaphors have to be stretched in order to accommodate exemplars such as alcoholism or David's drapetomania), the easier it is to show that our mappings are in fact metaphorical extensions, and the more obvious the social theories and values at play.

On the other hand, in the approach here, the category of disorder is not merely subjective or relativistic, and so goes beyond the critical emphasis on the fact that the category of disorder is bound to a particular cultural and historical context. Whether the mappings of disorder are valid for a particular exemplar is a matter that can be rigorously debated (Fulford *et al.*, 2006; Sadler, 2005; Schaffner, 1999); we can reasonably come to the conclusion, based on a consideration of our shared cognitive-affective maps of disorder, of our knowledge of medical science, and of the details of the specific cases, that Conrad ought to be viewed as suffering from a disorder (where the body is unbalanced, broken-down, etc.), whereas David is best understood as seeking freedom from slavery (with his mind balanced, working, etc.). Just as good scientists use a mixture of conceptual thinking, empirical data, and scientific values to make judgements about when to change their theories, so good nosology requires a range of considerations. However, insofar as categories are used in actions, they are subject to objective constraints, and so may be more or less right or wrong.

Although there will always remain controversy about what kinds of deviance are disorders, it should be emphasized that there is also a great deal of universal agreement about basic-level experiences and mappings such as pain, and of prototypical exemplars of disorder. Our shared cognitive-affective maps (which are in turn based on our sensorimotor and affective neurocircuits, and the interactions of the brain-mind with the natural and social world) are not merely subjective or relativistic, but can provide a reasonable way of delineating pain from other kinds of distress, or disorders (where the body is unbalanced, broken-down, etc.) from other types of deviance. As science progresses and our maps become more sophisticated and powerful, there is the promise of optimizing our categorization of more controversial exemplars of disorder; we may choose to continue to employ existing metaphors of disorder or to create entirely new mappings to characterize them more aptly.

Similarly, while the advent of novel medical interventions contributes to changing the boundaries of disorders, such changes can be debated rationally. Prior to the advent of cholesterol-lowering agents, rather high levels of cholesterol were defined as "normal". After the advent of studies which showed that cholestatins were useful in lowering cholesterol and preventing medical morbidity, the cut-off for "normal" cholesterol levels was lowered. Furthermore, with the lowered purchase cost of older cholestatins, and studies demonstrating that treatment of relatively low levels of cholesterol was cost-effective in preventing medical morbidity, the cut-off was again lowered. Similarly, in the psychiatric literature, while some have argued for the value of linking threshold for diagnosis to more conservative criteria such as treatment seeking (Narrow *et al.*, 2002), others have emphasized the need for lower diagnostic thresholds given the high morbidity associated with milder cases and given the existence of cost-effective interventions (Kessler *et al.*, 2003).[17] (Considerations about cost-efficiency need, of course, to be balanced with a range of other considerations, so as not to discriminate against patients who require more expensive treatments (Boyle & Callahan, 1995; Harris, 1987; Landman & Henley, 1998; Sabin & Daniels, 1994)).[18] The introduction of new psychiatric agents brings hope for addressing unmet needs, but at the same time may lead to the overexpansion of particular diagnostic constructs (Hudson & Pope, 1990; Slavney, 1991).

It is worth emphasizing that, in the approach here, the same principles of categorization apply to both the physical and the social worlds. However, in the physical sciences, there is a focus on the categories of the physical world, while in the human sciences there is a focus on the categories of our social world. There is a good deal of universal agreement about the nature of basic-level categories, whether physical (e.g. chairs) or social (e.g. pain). In contrast, there can be a great deal of controversy about more abstract physical categories (such as medical disorder) or human categories (such as psychiatric disorder). (More precisely, psychiatry involves both natural science and categories, as well as human science and categories – for this reason we refer in this volume to "psychiatric disorder" or "brain-mind disorder", rather than to mental disorder).[19]

---

[17] Implicit in this analysis, every disorder can be assessed using both categorical and dimensional constructs (Jablensky, 2005; Kessler, 2002; Zachar & Kendler, 2007).

[18] Landman and Henley note that cost is a complex concept which includes, for example, individual and social cost, material and emotional cost, and real and opportunity cost (Landman *et al.*, 1998). Johnson argues that a focus on cost-effectiveness involves a MORAL ARITHMETIC metaphor, which is at the heart of utilitarianism (Johnson, 1993).

[19] The question has been raised of what is mental about mental disorder (Brülde & Radovic, 2006)? The analysis here suggests that an answer lies in good part in understanding the graded structure of the category "disorder". We address ontological and epistemological aspects of the mind-body problem, which are also relevant to understanding this issue, in subsequent chapters.

Nevertheless, in both the physical and social realms, we can rationally debate whether specific exemplars are being aptly categorized (as involving an unbalanced, broken-down body or mind, as "mad" or as "bad", as "medical" or as "moral", etc.), and choose appropriate maps based on the scientific data and other considerations. Put in terms of the fact–value distinction, although facts and values cannot be divorced in the consideration of medical and psychiatric disorders (Canguilhem, 1966; de Beaufort *et al.*, 2000; Fulford, 1989; Fulford *et al.*, 2005; Hare, 1983; Pellegrino & Thomasma, 1981; Sadler, 1997, 2002; Schaffner, 1999; Wakefield, 1992b), we can rigorously assess these facts and values (Fulford *et al.*, 2006; Sadler, 2005; Schaffner, 1999). Hippocrates, Aristotle, and subsequent philosophers have emphasized that medicine is not only based on scientific knowledge (or episteme), but also that its arts and practices (or techne), involve practical reason and aim at the alleviation of human suffering (Gillett, 2006; Pellegrino, 1997; Simon, 1978); and clinical work can therefore be carefully weighed up.

As already noted, a range of authors have previously addressed the question of how to define medical and psychiatric disorder (Caplan *et al.*, 1981; Carson & Burns, 1997; Humber & Almeder, 1997; Sadler *et al.*, 1994); the approach here combines different aspects of two divergent positions (the classical and the critical). In line with an integrative perspective, it is notable that even Wakefield, who has rigorously pursued an essentialist view of disorder, agrees that disorders have an evaluative component, and admits that terms such as dysfunction have areas of vagueness, where boundaries are hard to define (Wakefield, 1999a). Conversely, Lilienfeld and Marino, who have denied a scientific basis for categorizing conditions as disorders, agree that at the heart of the idea of disorder is a breakdown, and admit that some disorders involve evolutionary dysfunction (Lilienfeld & Marino, 1999).

Thus, as Bolton (2000, 2008) points out, there is some convergence between these authors; Wakefield as well as Lilienfeld and Marino agree that in approaching mental disorder one needs (1) paradigm cases to guide one, and (2) a minimal theoretical core concerned with the idea that there is something wrong. We will return to these authors and their fascinating debate later on, when we consider explanatory accounts of disorders and their treatment. (Our argument will be that although evolutionary explanations – like other medical explanations – are important in understanding disorder and in considering claims that conditions are disorders, evolutionary theory does not itself provide necessary and sufficient criteria for the notion of "dysfunction", or that if there is an insistence on defining dysfunction in an essentialist way then such a construct does not fully capture current (valid and evaluative) understandings of disorder.)

A number of other authors have also emphasized prototypes, ideal types, or exemplars in the clinic (Blashfield *et al.*, 1985; Cantor *et al.*, 1980; Horowitz *et al.*, 1981; Jaspers, 1963; Livesley, 1985, 1986; Mezzich, 1989; Sadegh-Zadeh, 2005; Schaffner, 1994; Schwartz & Wiggins, 1987), or have attempted to provide a philosophical framework for clinical practice that draws on diverse theories and methods (Ghaemi, 2003; Hundert, 1989; Jaspers, 1963; Kriel, 2000; Matthews, 2004; McHugh & Slavney, 1988).[20] One well-known clinical model, based on systems theory, is the biopsychosocial approach, which emphasizes that psychiatric disorder involves multiple causal factors and which can therefore be accepted by those with quite varied views (Engel, 1977).[21] The current analysis makes a contribution by emphasizing that it is possible to simultaneously reject an essentialist view of disorders and also insist that altered function is underpinned by real embodied structures and mechanisms. This explains why some (more typical) disorders seem so easily explicable using classical terms, while other (more atypical) disorders seem to be explained by a different, more critical approach, and allows space for the development of a scientific psychiatric nosology which incorporates a carefully balanced view.

[20] Notably, much of this work has been driven by a critical concern with the limitations of a classical view of medicine, and in particular its focus on the body and its neglect of the person (Kriel, 2000; Schwartz & Wiggins, 1986), an issue we discuss later on (e.g. disease vs. illness).

[21] Instead of the term "biopsychosocial" (coined by Roy Grinker), I often use the term "psychobiological" (popularized by Adolf Meyer), to emphasize the increasing integration of the biological and the psychological, and the awareness that behaviour has to be understood both in terms of its overall meaning and underlying mechanism. We return to this issue below (e.g. explanations of pathogenesis and treatment).

Conclusion

The conceptual approach taken throughout the volume will follow the tack taken in the chapter. Thus, we will begin by outlining a classical approach that generally reflects the viewpoint of one or other philosopher within the analytic tradition. Then we will note the various critiques of such an approach that can be made. Finally, rather than attempt to resolve this debate on its own philosophical terms, we will ask, what can be concluded from the data of cognitive-affective science? Such data will generally reinforce a view that the mind-brain is embodied; sensorimotor and affective neuronal circuitry allows humans to interact with their physical and social world, and this in turn leads to the development of basic-level and abstract cognitive-affective maps (or metaphors) for understanding the world. The existence of such embodied structures and mechanisms is consistent with a realist position that draws on aspects of the classical position (e.g. its view that science is valid) and of the critical position (e.g. its scepticism about essentialism).

4

Conceptual questions about psychotropics

In this chapter we cover a series of questions about the nature of certain categories that are relevant to psychopharmacology. We have already developed a particular contrast within philosophy in the discussion of categories – the classical vs. critical approaches. The classical approach takes the view that words can mirror the categories of the world. The critical approach takes the view that categories are social constructs that reflect the subjectivity of a particular time and place. The synthetic or integrative position taken here says that categories strongly reflect the way in which the brain-mind interacts with the world, that this interaction is biologically grounded so contributing to the existence of minimal standards of agreement, and that it is possible to debate reasonably (that is, cognitive-affectively) their validity.

In the next sections this schema is used to discuss in turn, the nature of psychotropics, of emotion, and of the self. We could perhaps begin with any number of other constructs in philosophy of medicine and mind in order to reach similar conclusions, but these constructs are particularly relevant to the practice of psychopharmacology. The aim is not so much to defend the schema ("classical" vs. "critical"), which is an often over-simplifying framework on which to hang the different parts of this volume, but rather to put forward a conceptual position, based in part on cognitive-affective data, on a number of key concepts about medications/enhancements, about affective/cognitive phenomena, and about the persons/patients for whom we prescribe psychotropics in order to alter the brain-mind.

Medications, substances, neutraceuticals, and enhancements – what are the distinctions amongst psychotropics?

(A) *Abigail Adams recalled that during college she had managed to participate in social events by relying on alcohol. Just prior to going to a party, she would drink several sherries in her apartment. This helped her relax, and by the time she arrived at the party she would actually feel quite confident. She made a rule of not drinking any longer at parties; this was partly because she feared that if she had too much alcohol on board she would embarrass herself, and partly because she was aware that with too much alcohol she ran the risk of doing something really foolish.*

(B) *Abigail Adams read an article stating that inositol, a carbohydrate, is as effective for certain mood and anxiety disorders as marketed antidepressants. She did a literature search on the Internet, and learned that this agent has been shown effective for a number of conditions using rigorous randomized, placebo-controlled trials, of the sort in which she earlier participated. She liked the idea that inositol is a natural product and not a drug. She decided to discontinue her social anxiety disorder medication and instead to start taking inositol.*

(C) *An international athletics organization barred competitors from taking psychostimulants and steroids. A national coach, Ethan Endermann, instructed his team to take large doses of inositol on a daily basis. As this is simply a type of carbohydrate, there was no evidence from blood tests that an external agent had been administered. Nevertheless, the national team felt that they had increased energy and a more positive outlook on their game. An opposing team lodged a formal complaint against Endermann, charging that he had flouted the rules of the organization.*

Psychotropics – or brain-mind-altering substances – are used in a variety of contexts; it is important to distinguish medical therapies from substances of potential abuse (like alcohol), and ordinary nutrients (like inositol). In addition, a number of other distinctions are often required – between psychotropics that have been formally registered for use in particular psychiatric disorders, those that are "experimental", and drugs that are used for the purposes of "enhancement". Antidepressants are licensed as therapies for depression; in contrast, cocaine is classified as an addictive substance. Antidepressants are considered experimental for adult attention deficit/hyperactivity disorder, and might be thought of as an enhancement technology for certain disadvantageous character traits such as shyness.

The term "nootropic" (from the Greek noos for "mind", and tropein meaning "towards") has been used to describe cognitive-enhancing agents. An early professional literature used this term to describe medications that were employed to ameliorate the side-effects of electroconvulsive therapy. A more recent literature aimed at lay readers discusses the use of agents to enhance cognitive function (Dean *et al.*, 1993). A range of terms has similarly been used to describe the mood-enhancing properties of psychotropics, ranging from the professional "thymoleptic" to the lay "happy pill".

Terms such as "psychedelic" ("soul-revealing") and "entheogen" ("become divine within") have increasingly been used by those who promote the value of psychotropic drugs for spiritual or mystical purposes (Forte *et al.*, 2000; Ott & Hofmann, 1996; Wasson *et al.*, 1988). Empirical work on psychotropics as spiritual enhancers dates back several decades (Huxley, 1954; Pahnke, 1969).[1] In a recent rigorous study, volunteers given psilocybin reported the experience as having substantial personal meaning and spiritual significance, and as leading to sustained positive changes in attitudes and behaviour (Griffiths *et al.*, 2006).

Textbooks of biochemistry and neuroscience describe the endogenous chemical pathways in the body and brain. In contrast, textbooks of pharmacology and psychopharmacology cover a range of agents, describing how these exogenous compounds are taken up by the body and metabolized (pharmacokinetics), and how they affect receptors

---

[1] The physician-philosopher William James wrote about his experiences with nitrous oxide, concluding that there are many different forms of consciousness. The term "hallucinogen" was promoted by Huxley, who had participated in experiments by psychiatrist Humphry Osmond, who coined the word "psychedelic".

in the body (pharmacodynamics). This classical division of labour is consistent with a lay perspective that places a strict division between categories involving the body (and endogenous organic compounds) and those related to external objects (and exogenous synthetic compounds).

More classical authors have also attempted to provide necessary and sufficient criteria for distinguishing between therapies and "enhancements". It might also be argued that those drugs which are found effective in randomized controlled trials (RCTs) for the treatment of disease can be considered for registration as medication, and everything else should be considered "experimental". Sabin and Daniels (1994), relying on a classical conception of disorder as a functional impairment, argue that therapies are interventions which address disease, whereas enhancements merely improve human performance or appearance. In the USA, the cautions of the President's Council on Bioethics (2003) against enhancements implicitly accept the notion that these can readily be distinguished from treatments.

In contrast, the critical position is fond of interrogating distinctions between the natural and the unnatural. Social categorizations and distinctions between natural versus unnatural, or clean versus unclean (Douglas, 1984), say more about the culture and time at hand than about the reality of the world. Similarly, distinctions between "natural" and "unnatural" medications, or "clean" and "dirty" drugs, are socially constructed, rather than necessarily reflective of the particular properties of the relevant pharmaceuticals and psychotropics. Even the criteria that define "experimental" change from time to time and place to place: most selective serotonin reuptake inhibitors (SSRIs) are not yet formally registered as therapeutic agents in Japan.

From this perspective, the boundaries between the therapeutic, recreational, and enhancement use of drugs are highly permeable. Compounds like methylphenidate may be employed by conventional medicine (for the treatment of attention deficit/hyperactivity disorder) and by drug addicts (to obtain a high); conversely, a range of abused substances may have therapeutic potential. Severe shyness is characterized by significant overlap with social anxiety disorder and disability, thus using a medication to treat such symptoms can be validly seen either as therapeutic or as enhancement. Similarly, a consideration of the use of growth hormone for short stature suggests that the distinction between treatment and enhancement is porous (Allen & Fost, 1990). A bioethics report to the European Commission argued that there is no clear delineation between surgical treatment and enhancement (Bolt *et al.*, 2002).

What does cognitive-affective science say? There is not a great deal of literature in its sub-disciplines of cognitive psychology, artificial intelligence, linguistics, anthropology, developmental psychology, and philosophy that has tackled directly questions of how to differentiate different kinds of psychotropics. Nevertheless, in the course of this volume we have noted how cognitive-affective research is often inconsistent with both algorithmic approaches to categories (which may fail to capture the graded nature and social construction of concepts) and narrative approaches to categories (which may fail to capture the underlying structures and mechanisms that are able to provide a reasonable grounding of concepts, including those most relevant to the brain-mind). A detailed knowledge of the psychobiology of psychotropics may allow an integrated approach to conceptualizing their more objective or physical aspects (e.g. their mechanism of action) as well as their more subjective or socially constructed aspects (e.g. our experience of their actions).

The cognitive-affective sciences that have perhaps had the most to say about the distinctions between medications, substances, neutraceuticals, and enhancements, are neuroscience and evolutionary science. Neuroscience research has emphasized that registered medications and addictive substances associated with dependence and withdrawal tend to have structures that act on particular common brain-mind mechanisms, but there is not necessarily any such distinction in structure or mechanism between molecules that are manufactured in factories or extracted from herbs or foods, that are found endogenously or exogenously, that are formally licensed or not, or that are therapeutic versus enhancing.

An evolutionary perspective on the distinctions between psychotropics – focusing on distal survival mechanisms rather than proximal brain-mind mechanisms – may also be useful (Nesse & Berridge, 1997; Stein, 2006). Given our co-evolution with animal and plant species, it is not surprising that exogenous molecules are found endogenously (e.g., there are endogenous cannabinoids, which are the active ingredient of marijuana), or that endogenous and exogenous compounds both act via the same neuronal systems and receptors (e.g., SSRIs act at a very specific site – the serotonin reuptake pump, a protein that has evolved over millions of years and that ordinarily transports endogenous serotonin). Medications, substances, nutrients, and other kinds of psychotropics can have powerful brain-mind effects precisely because they affect complex, evolved, endogenous circuitry.

Work in cognitive psychology, connectionist modelling, and developmental science further contributes to understanding the mechanisms by which psychotropics act; for example, registered medications and addictive substances associated with dependence and withdrawal may lead to distinctive responses in particular paradigms. There is a growing literature on the anthropology of psychiatric medications (Lakoff, 2006), which contributes to understanding the real effects of classifying a particular agent as a medication, substance, or nutrient. For example, whether a particular psychotropic is conceptualized as a "mind-altering" medication, or as a "natural" herb may have significant effects on which patients are willing to consume it.

With these kinds of data and concepts in mind, we can return to our vignettes. It seems that psychobiological distinctions and overlaps amongst the psychotropics are not necessarily reflected in our social classifications. For example, registered medications and illegal substances that lead to symptoms of dependence both tend to act on particular brain circuits and related neurochemicals, and are associated with specific withdrawal symptoms when discontinued. Similarly, registered medications and herbs can have similar mechanisms of action; St. John's Wort is a herb with serotonin reuptake properties, but it blocks the serotonin reuptake pump with significantly less potency than do formally registered SSRIs.

In some ways the social distinctions noted in the vignettes can therefore be seen to be trivial. Inositol may be a carbohydrate, but when taken in large doses it is a psychotropic, with both positive therapeutic and negative adverse effects (Fux et al., 1996). The new term "neutraceutical" (Hardy et al., 2003) is in many ways apt. Many synthetic compounds were initially found in plants and herbs; the body and brain do not distinguish whether a compound is synthesized in a plant or in a factory. On the other hand, inositol is a particular kind of compound, dissimilar in its mechanism of action from performance-enhancing substances prohibited by sporting organizations (e.g. steroids), and so many would argue that it can be used by athletes legally and legitimately.[2]

The legal distinction between a formally registered medication and one that is prescribed "off-label" is also one that typically deserves not to be made too much of. A decision to attempt to register a drug for a particular licensed indication not only involves scientific decisions, but also marketing considerations. Thus a drug that is known to be effective for a particular medical or psychiatric disorder may not be registered because it is not profitable, at a particular time or in a particular place, to do this. Off-label use of medications, including psychotropics is, however, common – as always, the clinical decision-making process should be documented, in order to demonstrate an appropriate rationale.

However, some of the issues raised by the vignettes above are far from trivial. Many people may prefer "natural" herbal agents to factory-made ones; despite the fact that the relevant compounds may not be chemically distinguishable (LaFrance *et al.*, 2000). This preference helps fuel the huge "alternative medicines" industry or "indigenous medicines" industry, despite the fact that herbal agents, like synthetic ones, have both therapeutic and adverse effects, but are often not rigorously studied or regulated. Just as the psychotropics of the pharmaceutical industry require formal testing and licensing, so it would seem reasonable to argue that such standards should also apply to many of the compounds produced by alternative manufacturers (Wolfe, 2003).

Similarly, while certain psychotropics are primarily conceptualized and marketed as enhancers of recreation (including nicotine,

---

[2] Tamburrini (2006) argues that the essential purpose of sport is to expand the limits of our capacities, so that any kind of doping is acceptable. Brown (1984) earlier argued similarly. A contrasting argument is that modern athletics now must live with the costs of always wondering how much of performance is enhanced by such technology.

caffeine, alcohol) or performance (a range of molecules are advertised as increasing academic and sporting ability), the brain-behaviour effects (whether positive or negative) of such molecules deserve serious consideration. Early on, tobacco was touted as having performance-enhancing benefits; it took several decades for nicotine to be recognized as an addictive substance and cigarette-smoking as harmful (Pennock, 2007). Today, the alcohol industry promotes the health benefits of red wine, but there is also clear evidence of individual and social harms associated with drinking.

For this volume, the crucial distinction between different kinds of psychotropics, or different uses of psychotropics, is that between treatment and enhancement. If there is no distinction between the structure of therapeutic and enhancing psychotropics, or in the mechanisms on which they act, a cognitive-affective perspective might then conceivably try to distinguish validly between the prototypic scenarios in which treatment and enhancement are prescribed. If treatment is prescribed in response to disorder, while enhancements are provided by those in the recreational and sporting industries, this would have normative implications for health care professionals (treatments should be offered, enhancements need not be; Sabin & Daniels, 1994).

However, we earlier emphasized that definitions of disorder are porous. The more common and disabling a "disorder", and the more effective and inexpensive a relevant molecule, the more likely we are to want to justify its use in "treatment". Interventions such as routine vaccination and fluoride supplementation are no longer thought of as "enhancement", even though they are preventive measures that were only introduced relatively recently. In other cases, boundaries are much more difficult to decide (in some cases of social anxiety, the use of a psychotropic could be defined as a treatment, and in other cases as an enhancement). Good judgement is therefore required for individual clinical decisions. The following two chapters provide additional discussion (on explanatory questions, and on ethical issues) relevant to coming to such a judgement. We must first, however, address some other conceptual questions relevant to psychopharmacology.

Psychotropics for personality – what is emotion?

Abigail Adams decided to participate in the research testing a new medica-
tion for the treatment of social anxiety disorder. By the end of the clinical
trial she felt a different person. In particular, she was more confident in
social situations. This in turn made her feel less worried about life and
more able to enjoy things in general. At work things gradually started to go
more smoothly, and after a few more months she was given a promotion.
At about that time she came to the conclusion: I did have a disorder, what I
thought of as "shyness" was in fact a definite disability. She had read about
Hippocrates' classification of temperament, and decided that she had had
a disordered temperament.

The classical approach to science and language, as noted in the previous chapter, leads to particular views of mind and of medicine, and
of categories such as emotion and personality. Although linguistic-
analytic philosophers have only more recently begun to pay attention
to emotion,[3] the nature of emotion has long been of substantial interest to philosophy, with a classical view often emphasizing the formal
components of emotion, and arguing that any specific emotion can be
characterized in terms of particular beliefs and desires. An emphasis
on the logical aspects of emotion has gone together with a tendency
to ignore feeling (including bodily feeling) as part of emotion, and to
overlook the links between emotion and character traits.

The emphasis in the classical position on the importance of the
rational has arguably gone hand in hand with a devaluation of emotion –
philosophers from Plato (2003) to Descartes (1650) and Kant (1781)
have contrasted reason with passion, typically favouring the former
faculty.[4] An early view contrasted bodily emotion, with the abstract
realm of reason. More recent views continue to put emotion to one

---

[3] A range of authors have contributed to this literature (Ben-Ze'ev, 2000; Blackburn, 1998;
Gibbard, 1990b; Goldie, 2000; Golsling, 1965; Greenspan, 1988; Hatzimoysis, 2003; Kenny,
1963; Langer, 1942; Lyon, 1980; Neu, 1977; Prinz, 2004; Roberts, 2003; Rorty, 1980;
Solomon, 2004; Stocker & Hegeman, 1992; Thalberg, 1977).

[4] The Stoics and the Epicureans are particularly critical of the emotions as irrational; for
them, philosophy serves as therapy, ensuring the soul is purged of such vagaries.

side; a philosophical view of emotions as primarily involving beliefs and desires has been termed cognitivism, and within psychology schools influenced by the classical position – behaviourism and symbolic cognitivism – have also often downplayed affective phenomena per se. Thus symbolic cognitivists' view of the mind as a computational transformer means that emotion is conceptualized merely as a cognition interrupter or as a type of information (Le Doux, 1996), and subjective feeling is replaced with a marker of the intensity of emotion.

Within the classical perspective, it makes sense to classify abnormalities of emotion in distinctive categories (e.g. anxiety disorders, mood disorders), and to define these in terms of necessary and sufficient characteristics; this is the approach of nosological systems such as the American Psychiatric Association's Diagnostic and Statistical Manual (DSM) (American Psychiatric Association, 1994). The emphasis in defining diagnostic criteria for these disorders is on objective observable criteria, rather than on subjective hard-to-define feelings. Thus social anxiety disorder (SAD) is listed on axis I of DSM-IV, within the category of anxiety disorders, and is characterized by symptoms of anxiety triggered in particular social contexts.

From this perspective, it would similarly be reasonable to use pharmacological interventions to reverse abnormalities of emotion, perhaps by altering desires. However, the link between emotion, character, and their embodiment in the brain-mind, may be overlooked. Thus, in DSM-IV, avoidant personality disorder (APD), which is characterized by a pervasive pattern of social inhibition, feelings of inadequacy in social situations, and hypersensitivity to negative evaluation, and therefore shares many features of social anxiety disorder, is nevertheless listed on axis II together with other disorders of personality. Furthermore, whereas studies of axis I disorders have tended to focus on medication, most studies of anxiety II disorders, such as avoidant personality disorder, have tended to focus on psychotherapy.

A critical view of science and language leads to an entirely different approach to psychology in general, and to emotion and its disorders in particular. First, emotions cannot be specified in formal terms: they have porous boundaries with one another (Sartre, 1948), and they are intentional – they involve feelings towards objects in the world (Goldie,

2000; Helm, 2001) and so must be understood within particular contexts. Any attempt to reduce human behaviours and feelings to universal categories – whether in the Hippocratic system or in DSM – is inherently problematic; instead we should attempt to delineate how emotions are constructed by societies in different ways, at different times and places (Hacker, 2004; Harré, 1986b), and conversely, how moods connect the self to the world and are world-constitutive (Heidegger, 1962; Svenaeus, 2007).

Second, feeling (including bodily feeling) is very much part of emotion. Indeed, this subjective aspect of emotion makes it resistant to purely scientific inquiry or computational modelling, but also is what makes it so uniquely important. Indeed, on the critical view, emotional experience is superior to cold reason; emotions not only shape and determine what we value, but may be an important end in themselves. Although Plato might be said by many to have a more classical view of emotion, the Phaedrus notes that "the greatest goods come to men through madness"(Plato, 2003). Insofar as emotion is understood within the narrative of a person's life, there is also a strong link between emotion and character, with some dispositions being "deeper" than others (Morton, 1980).

These critical positions then have implications for understanding social anxiety. First, the overlap between social anxiety and normality may be emphasized; there are no fixed boundaries between normal variation and psychiatric disorder – rather this latter category reflects cultural and historical theories and values. It may be argued that the idea that shyness was a social anxiety disorder gained popularity only after it was proposed by those with a biologically influenced construction of psychiatry, and given particular impetus by a pharmaceutical industry attempting to increase the market for antidepressant products. This claim about "disease mongering" has been made for a range of psychiatric conditions (Degrandpre, 2006; Healy, 2004; Kutchins & Kirk, 1997; McHenry, 2006; Moynihan & Henry, 2006; Starcevic, 2002; Szasz, 2001; Valenstein, 1998), including social anxiety disorder (Lane, 2007; Moynihan, 2002; Moynihan & Smith, 2002).

It makes more sense, from a critical perspective, to view social anxiety in terms of a person's experience of the world and their characteristic ways of feeling and of responding. Rather than being reified as a disorder, social anxiety may represent a valuable response to and an authentic feeling in a world where social relationships are characterized by threat (Glas, 2004; Kierkegaard, 1981; Small, 1984). Variations in emotional experience, in character traits, and in our personal narratives, have been medicalized; another example of the way in which psychiatry has intruded into our lives and exerted increasing control over our thoughts and feelings. This medicalization of emotional experience should be strongly resisted.

What do the data from cognitive-affective science say? A range of data indicate, first, that emotion and character, contra the classical approach, cannot be reduced to a formal algorithm and are inextricably linked with reason; and, second, that emotion and character, contra the critical approach, are not merely socially constructed, but have universal elements that can be understood in terms of the brain-mind, and its activity within the world. This third position, integrating objective and subjective aspects of emotion, is consistent with a realist and embodied position in psychology, and with a view in psychiatry that, first, psychotropics can lead to changes in emotion and personality; and, second, that the advantages and disadvantages of this change can reasonably be weighed.[5] To reach this conclusion, a range of cognitive-affective science data from different disciplines is briefly covered.

Cognitive psychology has increasingly come to the conclusion that cognition and emotion structure one another, and so are inextricably linked (Damasio, 1994; Greenberg & Safran, 1991; Hamilton *et al.*, 1988; James, 1890; Miller *et al.*, 1960; Oatley & Johnson-Laird, 1987; Power & Dalgleish, 1997; Schulkin, 2004).[6] As Hume (1739), Spinoza (1677), and others recognized, reason cannot easily be divorced from

---

[5] The objective and subjective components of emotion are emphasized in the clinical differentiation between affect (transient and objective emotional state) and mood (sustained and subjective emotional tone) (Selby, 2003).

[6] James (1884) put forward the "peripheralist" idea that emotion follows our responses to arousing stimuli (a position that has influenced Damasio's somatic marker hypothesis (Damasio, 1994)). Cannon (1927) took a centralist position, emphasizing that emotions arise from cognitive appraisal of emotional stimuli. Today, there is growing rapprochement between these positions (Morris, 2002).

passion. Thus, it is sensible to respect our emotional responses and to listen carefully to what they say. Furthermore, it is not simply the case that emotion leads to cognition, or cognition to emotion; rather, these phenomena occur in parallel (Greenberg & Safran, 1991).

The question of how best to model emotion in computational terms is a difficult one (Picard, 1997; Rey, 1980). Nevertheless, current work in this area does not attempt to reduce emotion to a simple algorithm (Arbib & Fellous, 2004). Instead, there is an effort to describe particular emotions as emerging from the interaction of a particular agent with its environment, and to recognize the value of dissecting out the unique physiological embodiment of cognition-emotion.[7] As Wittgenstein (1967) pointed out in the *Investigations*, emotional states are inextricably embedded in "the stream of life"; we cannot locate them as fixed or universal forms, rather we must consider how they are used in particular social situations (see, for example, the earlier quotation from Harrison about pain). Thus emotion emerges from a particular configuration of the brain-mind, and its experience in the world.

Neuroscientific data are consistent with a view that emphasizes a porous boundary between cognition and emotion. Although prefrontal circuits play an important role in cognition, and subcortical circuits play an important role in emotion, the different regions of the brain are closely and continuously interlinked (Davidson, 2003; Dolan, 2002; Le Doux, 1996; Panksepp, 1998). Specific lesions may result in the apparent dissociation of emotional and cognitive processing, but in ordinary circumstances they inter-relate seamlessly (Damasio, 1994, 2003). Neuroscientific data also reinforce that emotion and character are mediated by the brain-mind, with a growing database of studies on the neuronal circuitry and molecular mechanisms that underpin affect and personality. Different emotions do not simply reduce to different circuitry (Kagan, 2006); for example, the amygdala seems important in modulating memory for events according to emotional importance, regardless of whether the emotion is pleasant or aversive (Hamann *et al.*, 1999). Nevertheless, regions of the brain that monitor the state of

---

[7] There is also the view that in order to succeed in certain kinds of tasks, computers must be emotional in some way (Delancey, 2001; Minsky, 2006; Picard, 1997).

the body – creating body maps – are particularly important in mediating feelings (Damasio, 1994, 2003).

Linguistic data confirm that the particular psychobiological under-pinnings of emotion have led to a universality of emotional experi-ence – the metaphors and mappings of emotion cut across history and geography, and prototypic emotions are therefore widely understood (de Sousa, 1987; Griffiths, 1997; Kovecses, 1986; Russell, 1991). Lakoff (1987), for example, describes how anger is universally structured in terms of a specific set of metaphors and mappings, drawn from the subjective feelings and bodily changes that occur during this emotion. Across different times and cultures, anger will be described as "hot" rather than "cool", as "explosive" rather than as "contained" (Braund & Most, 2004). As Williams James pointed out in his classical paper, "What is an emotion": "A purely disembodied human emotion is a nonentity".

At the same time, the brain-mind operates within different social contexts which may structure the experience of emotion in different ways (Elster, 1999a, b; Walton, 2004). Evolutionary, developmental, and anthropological data confirm a view of brain-mind operating accord-ing to universal mechanisms, but within particular contexts. Emotions have long-standing evolutionary value and therefore several universal characteristics (Darwin, 1965). Modern evolutionary science is increas-ingly able to put forward data-based hypotheses about the origins and structure of various emotions (Buss, 2005; Nesse, 1990), including their value in rational decision-making (Evans & Cruse, 2004; Frank, 1988). Insofar as complex emotions are mediated by phylogenetically ancient mechanisms, evolutionary science provides an important perspective on the embodiment of emotion (explaining, for example, links between the psychobiology of physical pain, and the pain of social exclusion (Panksepp, 2003)). During human ontological development, however, emotions are structured somewhat differently from time to time, and place to place (Gordon, 1987). Developmental and cross-cultural psy-chologists are increasingly able to describe the gradual maturation of cognitive and emotional structures, as well as the variation of such structures across individuals and across communities.

Conceptual work in philosophy also supports the integrative approach to emotion taken here. First, philosophers from at least as far back as Aristotle (1984) have noted that emotions can be reasonable (or appropriate and proportional) or not (de Sousa, 1987; Hume, 1739; Nussbaum, 2001; Smith, 2002; Solomon, 1993). Emotions develop within certain contexts, so the person who is subjected to child abuse learns distrust of people; but while such an emotion or character is understandable, it may no longer be adaptive or appropriate. Contra a critical view that over-emotionalizes affect; there are degrees with which one can be reflectively aware of one's own emotions and their triggers and consequences, and while culture may inform decisions about the appropriateness of emotions such decisions are also open to reasoned (including passionately reasoned) debate. Second, philosophers have emphasized the embodiment of emotion, noting the close relation between passion and reason, between emotion and bodily feeling (Wollheim, 1999), between emotion and action in the world (Goldie, 2000), and even the changes in the embodiment of emotion after pharmacotherapy (Svenaeus, 2007). Contra a classical view that over-intellectualizes emotion, emotion is not simply an add-on to beliefs and desires, nor can emotion be understood as existing outside of its brain-mind and interpersonal context.

In addition to these general concepts and data from the cognitive-affective sciences on emotion, there is a growing body of research on social anxiety in particular. Social anxiety and related traits such as behavioural inhibition are characterized by particular kinds of cognitions and affects, as well as by particular neuronal and molecular features (Schwartz *et al.*, 2003). While some people with behavioural inhibition manage fine, others develop social anxiety later in life (Kagan *et al.*, 1988). Such social anxiety takes place in prototypic contexts (that cannot be formally specified in terms of necessary and sufficient criteria), is underpinned by the brain-mind and its experience of the world, and is open to rigorous debate about whether it is appropriate or whether it should be medically treated. Although there is debate about whether social anxiety disorder represents an evolutionary-based adaptive response (Wakefield *et al.*, 2005) or a biologically based "false alarm" (Stein & Bouwer, 1997), there is general agreement that people with the symptoms of this condition suffer distress and have functional impairment (Campbell-Sills & Stein, 2005).

If (contra the classical view) we accept the view from cognitive-affective science that emotions cannot simply be specified in terms of formal and distinct categories, then the division between normal social anxiety, shyness, and social anxiety disorder may not be found "in nature". In the past, those interested in biological psychiatry and psychopharmacological interventions focused primarily on DSM axis I disorders, while those interested in personality, psychodynamics and psychotherapy focused on DSM axis II disorders. But the symptoms of social anxiety disorder and the traits of avoidant personality disorder show a good deal of overlap (Schneier *et al.*, 2002), both fall along dimensions of severity, it is not clear that they are mediated by different structures and mechanisms, and both may respond to similar kinds of pharmacotherapy and psychotherapy (Deltito & Stam, 1989; Muller *et al.*, 2004). Thus, the contrast between social anxiety disorder and avoidant personality disorder may not have a great deal of clinical utility.

If (contra the critical view) we accept that the view from cognitive-affective science that emotions are mediated by the brain-mind and are an essential component of reasoning validly about the world then it is not surprising that psychotropic interventions change not only emotional states (classified on DSM axis I) but also character traits (classified on DSM axis II) in a useful way. In particular, it would not be surprising that particular medications therefore decrease feelings of social anxiety, and diminish personality traits of social avoidance. Similar kinds of consideration apply to other personality disorders, where there is growing appreciation of their underpinnings by specific kinds of neuroanatomical and neurochemical findings, and increasing use of pharmacotherapeutic interventions (Cloninger, 1987; Siever & Davis, 1991). Just as there is no fault line in nature between disorder and non-disorder, so in considering particular categories of disorder, including social anxiety disorder (Muller *et al.*, 2004), it is notable that their characteristic emotional symptoms typically fall along dimensions (Jablensky, 2005; Kessler, 2002; Zachar & Kendler, 2007).

The position here emphasizes that emotion is not entirely socially constructed and relativistic; it is possible to debate rationally (cognitively-emotionally) as to whether a particular emotion is appropriate or not, and whether interventions to alter emotional experience are appropriate or not. Boundaries between normal social anxiety, shyness, and social anxiety disorder can be validly determined (Stein, 1996b; Stein *et al.*, 1994), using considerations such as the nature of the underlying psychobiology, the presence of associated distress and impairment, and the availability of effective and cost-effective interventions (Ballenger *et al.*, 1998). The introduction of specific kinds of pharmacotherapy and psychotherapy that are able to normalize the neuroanatomical and neurochemical mechanisms that mediate social anxiety, and to lead to a significant reduction in these symptoms (Furmark *et al.*, 2002), is a welcome development, and it behoves clinicians to diagnose and treat people, like Abigail Adams, who suffer from social anxiety disorder or from particularly severe avoidant personality traits.

The psychobiology of self-representation – what is the self?

Reflecting on her experience several months after treatment, Abigail Adams came to the conclusion not merely that she suffered from a disordered temperament, but that she had now found her "true self". Before she took medication, she told her husband, she was only able to be genuinely spontaneous in his company. But now she could be her true self with everyone. She loved the fact that now when she walks into the office at work, she was able to offer a cheery "Good morning!" to everyone in sight. Before she was unable to do this, but only because of her shyness, and not because she didn't really want to be able to do this.

How can personal identity be defined, what is the true self?[8] A classical approach might suggest that personhood is determinate, with necessary

---

[8] Philosophy of personal identity has addressed a range of different questions including those about transfer of psychological life from one body to another (i.e. how can continuity of a living entity be defined), changes in personal identity over time (i.e. how can continuity of persons or selves be identified), authenticity and autonomy of the self (e.g. are one's thoughts and emotions truly expressive of who one is), and nature of personhood (e.g. to what extent does a fetus have the status of a person). For the purposes of drawing a broad conceptual contrast, these are to some extent conflated here. A partly related philosophy of "theory of mind", focused on understanding not the self but the other, will not be directly addressed.

and sufficient characteristics, and clear boundaries. Such a view has roots in a Platonic concept of the soul (Simon, 1978). Descartes, for example, argued that personal identity inheres in a Pure Ego or spiritual substance (Descartes, 1993). Kant refined this viewpoint, putting forward a transcendental idea of the self, a primordial and unified ego, which cannot appear in the boundaries of space and time (Kant, 1977). A series of philosophers, including some with an interest in psychiatric disorders, have subsequently attempted to provide more precise and accurate accounts of persons, selves, and related constructs.[9]

A classical approach might also try to identify persons or selves with the brain, the mind, or their experiences (Le Doux, 2002; Quinton, 1962).[10] Locke, having rejected the idea that personal identity resides in a spiritual substance, famously suggested that experience-memory is the defining characteristic of persons over time (Locke, 1694). He disentangled this notion of personal identity from the brain, arguing that experience-memory could be transplanted onto another body. Others have argued, however, that neurophysiological facts are key in understanding personal identity; for example, data that emerge from split-brain studies require a reconceptualization of the self (Nagel, 1989).

A classical approach to persons tends to be associated with a view of the self that emphasizes its unitary, conscious, and rational aspects, and that tends not to emphasize change in the self over time. This position leads to a certain kind of view within psychology, where the self can be neatly defined, perhaps in terms of a particular role that it plays within the mind. Similarly, in thinking about psychopathology, the idea of the self emerging only after the prescription of medication would likely seem counter-intuitive from this perspective. A classical position would more readily consider exemplars of a person taking a substance of abuse, like alcohol; here the person might, for example, ultimately be excused

---

[9] A range of authors have contributed to this literature (Atkins, 2005; Dennett, 1991; Fletcher, 1975; Glover, 1988; Goldie, 2004; Heginbotham, 2000; Lewis, 1983; Mackie, 1976; Martin, 1998; McGinn, 1983; Perry, 1975; Radden, 1996; Rorty, 1975; Schechtman, 1996; Seigel, 2005; Strawson, 1977, 1997; Taylor, 1989; Wilkes, 1988; Williams, 1994; Wollheim, 1984).

[10] The identification of self (or mind) with brain has been termed "neuroscientific essentialism" (Garland, 2004).

from acts committed after consuming alcohol (Locke, 1694); insofar as they acted out of character.[11]

A critical approach to persons and selves might, on the other hand, emphasize the difficulty in defining personal identity in any determinate way – the self is decentred, multiple, and malleable, and cannot be specified in terms of a formal algorithm. An emphasis on the decentred self has been a central feature of continental philosophy and of psychoanalysis (Elliott, 2001; Hansen & Maynes, 2005; Henriques *et al.*, 1984). Freud noted that,

There are cases in which parts of a person's own body, even portions of his mental life – his perceptions, thoughts and feelings – appear alien to him and as not belonging to his ego; there are other cases in which he ascribes to the external world things that clearly originate in his own ego and that ought to be acknowledged by it. Thus even the feeling of our own ego is subject to disturbances and the boundaries of the ego are not constant. (Freud, 1961)

More ordinarily, events such as physical disorder disrupt the self, threatening to make us different persons (Zaner, 1981).

A critical perspective may emphasize that the self is a fiction, which cannot simply be reduced to the physical continuity of the brain, nor to the psychological continuity of the mind. Hume (1739) argued that the self consists of a bundle of impressions strung together by the imagination, and so is a useful fiction for ordering our perceptions. Similarly, William James denied that there was any single entity at the core of the self that could be called an "I" – we experience ourselves as unified beings only on the basis of our passing states of consciousness. A range of philosophers have since explored the self in terms of narrative (Dennett, 1991; MacIntyre, 1981; Phillips, 2003; Ricoeur, 1992; Taylor, 1989; Velleman, 2006). The idea of the individual may have roots in Greek philosophy, but it is essentially a modern Western construct (Giddens, 1991; Morris, 1973), and modern technologies, including psychotherapy or psychotropics, should not be seen as enabling progress

---

[11] Locke's position is more complex than the classical approach sketched here. He is well aware of changes in persons over time, and understands that persons are self-constituting (Schechtman, 1996). His view about punishing drunkards is also complex; while God may excuse alcohol-induced behaviour, it is just for man to inflict punishment.

(Fukuyama, 2002) or as helping to determine the "true self" (Crossley, 2003; Elliott, 2003; Murray, 2007; Rose, 1998a, 2007), but rather should be understood as allowing social discipline (Martin *et al.*, 1988) or control (Deleuze, 1995). Foucault, for example, argues that whereas for the Greeks medicine was an instantiation of the "technology of life" (or "how to live the good life"), it has increasingly become a "technology of the self" (providing the very terms of the self; Martin *et al.*, 1988; Murray, 2007).

A critical approach to persons tends to be associated with a view that emphasizes the self as fractured, unconscious, and irrational, and this leads to particular views within psychology and psychopathology. Certainly, since Freud, it has also been difficult to accept people's view of their own selves without scepticism. While a critical perspective might accept the idea that medication is useful in experiencing one aspect of our selves, it is unlikely to accept any particular articulation of the self as necessarily more valid. Whereas a classical view typically characterizes behaviour on substances as "out of character", a critical view might emphasize the value of such experience, referring to the therapeutic importance of "mind-altering substances" or to the right to use drugs for recreational purposes (Husak, 1992). Indeed, a strand of antipsychiatry has opposed the use of psychotropics, but encouraged the use of substances of abuse (Ingleby, 1981; Sedgwick, 1982).

What do the cognitive-affective science data say? A range of data indicate, first, that personal identity, contra the classical approach, cannot be specified in terms of unchanging necessary and sufficient characteristics; and second, that personal identity, contra the critical approach, is not merely a social construction, but can be understood in terms of the brain-mind, and its experience within and of the world. Selves are embodied in the brain-mind, they are constructed within the narratives provided by social interaction, they are multidimensional and they change over time (Bermúdez *et al.*, 1995; Churchland, 2002; Flanagan, 1998; Sellars, 1963; Varela *et al.*, 1991). This third position is consistent with a realist and embodied position in psychology, and with a view in psychopharmacology that, first, psychotropics can lead to a change in the self, and, second, that the advantages and disadvantages of this change can reasonably be weighed. To reach this conclusion, we will briefly cover a range of data from cognitive-affective science.

Cognitive psychology has contributed a series of studies on self-awareness, self-recognition, and self-schemas (Harter, 1999; Leary & Tangney, 2002; Snodgrass & Thompson, 1997). A minimal sense of self emerges from our concrete perceptions and movements, while a sense of personal identity with continuity over time is enabled by and mediated through more abstract narrative (Bruner, 1990; Gallagher, 2000; Metzinger, 2003; Neisser, 1988; Neisser & Fivush, 1994). Such views are to some extent consistent with Hume's argument that the self consists of a bundle of impressions strung together by the imagination, and so is a useful fiction for ordering our perceptions (Hume, 1739). Like other schemas, self-schemas are only partial, and are subject to error. Personal awareness is certainly quite different from our knowledge of others, but a wholly introspectionist position is incorrect; any first-person reporting of mental states is fallible insofar as it may conflict with the person's actual actions (Goleman, 1996; Leary, 2006; Wegner, 2002).

Artificial intelligence work on robots operating within particular contexts has increasingly attempted to specify how top-down processes (modelling of the world) and bottom-up sensorimotor processes (representing environmental contexts) interact to structure the self (Gallagher, 2000). In one example, a robot modeller has argued that the self comes into existence when, in response to outside demands, the relationship between top-down and bottom-up processes becomes incoherent (Tani, 1998); this kind of approach is consistent with a view of the self as embodied, interactively constructed, and impermanent.[12]

Language and narrative play a crucial role in the development of selves and persons (Erchak, 1992; Harré, 1983; Leary & Tangney, 2002; Neisser *et al.*, 1991). Linguistic and anthropological data indicate that in the West and elsewhere, one common mapping of the self contrasts the Essential Self (the "true self") with a Second Self (not "true") which is incompatible with the Essential Self, and which is conceptualized as either a person or a container the first self hides in (Lakoff & Johnson,

---

[12] Sheryl Turkle has noted how the introduction of computing and the Internet has made it easier to understand the notion of the decentred self (Turkle, 2004).

1999). As Merleau-Ponty (1962) pointed out, we make sense of the world from the perspective of the body; even our concept of the self therefore necessarily has the character of an oriented space. This standard map of the self is similar in important ways to the classical view of self as unitary and rational, and allows us to reach conclusions of the form used by Abigail; namely, "I have found my true self".

Neuroscience data confirm the embodiment of the self in the brainmind (Feinberg & Keenan, 2005; Kircher & David, 2003; Le Doux, 2002; Mishara, 2007). A basic level of self-processing involves sensory integrative functions of the sort carried out by the parietal lobes, while more complex self-processing involves interaction of the inferior frontal cortex and the superior parietal lobe (Damasio, 1999). Affect likely plays a key role in the basic sense of self (Panksepp, 2005). A developed sense of self appears to be underpinned by the right hemisphere (Feinberg, 2001; Keenan *et al.*, 2001), while the left hemisphere plays a crucial role in generating narratives about the self (Gazzaniga, 1998). Although lesion and imaging studies cannot reduce selves to brain circuits (Dumit, 2004), they are leading to specific hypotheses about the anatomic bases of self-processing and self-monitoring (Decety & Sommerville, 2003; Northoff *et al.*, 2006). Similarly, substance abuse and other neuropsychiatric disorders can also precipitate depersonalization, allowing study of the neurochemical basis of selfhood (Hobson, 2001; Stephens & Graham, 2000). Again, while the self is far more than the genome, neurogenetics is gradually contributing to understandings of individual differences (Parens, 2004).

Developmental and evolutionary data confirm a view of the self as embodied in the brain-mind and in interpersonal interaction, as constructed, and as malleable. Studies of infants have indicated considerable cognitive-affective sophistication, suggesting that at birth there is a minimal self that is embodied and interactive (Rochat, 1995). Over time, through cognitive (Gopnik *et al.*, 1999; Piaget, 1952) and emotional (Schore, 1994; Stern, 2000) interaction with the world, the self becomes increasingly structured. In parallel, there is growing evidence of a minimal self in non-human primates, with evolution eventually allowing the development of more complex narrative selves when human brain-minds are situated in human groups. The self is not merely socially constructed or spiritual; our mapping capacities are evolution's extensions and elaborations of the rudimentary self rooted in somatosensory and autonomic systems (Churchland, 2002; Gallagher, 2000; Lakoff *et al.*, 1999; Varela *et al.*, 1991).

Philosophy confirms a view of the self as constructed and malleable, but also as embodied. Persons need to be understood both as objects (with crucial biological underpinnings), and as subjects (intentional agents with thoughts and emotions) (Schechtman, 1996). If we are to define the nature of a person – it would be, following Merleau-Ponty, as "an auto-constitution" – a being that is structured but that also constructs, with the structures that define and limit man's potentialities at the same time ensuring that personhood cannot be restricted to a fixed set of categories (van Niekerk, 1986). In addition, the standard metaphoric mapping of the Essential Self is flawed; as Hume (1739) suggested, persons are similar to clubs or nations; they exist, but over time, as their membership changes, the cut-offs between the old entity and the new entity become impossible to define. Even our notion of the self as the centre of a unique and private self-consciousness may well be a reflection of current discourse (Rorty, 1979). A range of thought experiments have contemplated persons being changed trait by trait, or neuron by neuron (often by a callous neurosurgeon); these show that there is no specific cut-point at which one person becomes another; personal identity lies on a continuum (Parfit, 1984), and there are degrees of personhood (Perring, 1997a). Finally, as both Hume and Merleau-Ponty noted, the self does not exist apart from the body. Philosophers have since continued to emphasize that the interpretation and organization of experience is always mediated through a body that is embedded in the world (Churchland, 2002; Legrand, 2006; Radden, 1996; Strawson, 1974; Thornton, 2003; van Niekerk, 1986).

In addition, we can reasonably consider whether some of our potential selves are better or worse than others (White, 1991). If we think about persons, contra a classical approach, not as immutable natural kinds, but rather as clubs with fuzzy boundaries, this has implications for our thoughts about changing them. For example, Parfit concludes that by treating people as nations, we adopt a more utilitarian approach (thus, we might not want to prioritize helping people who have previously suffered, but rather aim at relieving as much suffering as possible; Parfit, 1984). Similarly, if we think of persons as clubs, it may change our perspective on interventions that result in changes. When we make a change to a natural kind, this is necessarily drastic, because it becomes a different kind. But when we make a marked change to a club – for example, altering its uniform – the consequences may be less all-or-nothing.

Furthermore, contra an entirely subjective or relativistic approach to personal identity and selves, there are justifiable reasons for preferring some selves to others. Sadler (2003) has noted a "self-illness ambiguity", a fundamental blurring of personal self and psychiatric illness which leads to a metaphor not of "having a sickness" but of "being sick". Such new selves can be judged as better or as worse. People with schizophrenia may be viewed as experiencing the world in a uniquely creative way (the argument of antipsychiatry), or as being-in-the-world in a way that is ultimately impoverishing (the argument of most clinicians). Of course, a person with schizophrenia may make a correct or incorrect assessment about the extent to which their self-during-treatment is an improvement. But even if both clinician and patient agree that there is an overall improvement, the patient may feel some sense of loss of personal identity on treatment; the self-illness ambiguity creates ambivalence about treatment (Sadler, 2003).

With this conceptual framework in place, we can now return to Abigail. A person with social anxiety disorder may interact in the world in an entirely different way after successful pharmacological treatment, and it is therefore unsurprising that they experience this in terms of a new self. By altering the neurocircuitry underpinning the relevant systems, psychotropics may well influence abstract self-representational capacities and cognitive-affective maps. The standard metaphor of illness may not easily apply here, because there is not simply a response by the self to an external threat or obstacle, but rather there is a change in self. Indeed, when we consider aspects of identity the line between normal variation and pathology is often fuzzy (Elliott, 1999). Conversely, while the metaphor that the Essential Self has been changed or found may be used, selves are complex phenomena, even the concept of an authentic self is a self-narrative, and we need to think very carefully, using appropriately rigorous concepts, about the potential benefits and costs of treatment. "Technologies of the self" should not simply be seen as an advance, nor necessarily viewed as problematic, but they need to be carefully assessed and evaluated.[13]

In subsequent chapters, we will go beyond the focus here on categories, considering also explanatory and ethical issues, in order to be able to consider fully such benefits and costs. In the interim, it can be briefly noted that there may be good reasons for viewing Abigail as experiencing life as more authentic on treatment (e.g., she has less fear, and more options), and for characterizing people who are addicted to substances as experiencing inauthentic selves (e.g., they have more dysphoria, and their options are more restricted).[14] Although social anxiety disorder is a relatively new diagnosis and its treatments only recently developed, there may be underlying psychobiological mechanisms that account for the disorder, and which cut across time and place (we can point to historical figures who suffered from this disorder, and who recognized the significant limitations that this caused them). Furthermore, we can interview people with social anxiety disorder before and after treatment, and assess the way in which their symptoms decrease, or in which their lives have been enriched (in the clinical context, a judgement of improvement requires both medical knowledge and empathic skills).

What of the fact that Abigail did not originally regard herself as having a disorder? What of the fact that even though we may not believe in the concept of a true self, Abigail does? It is relevant to note that cognitive-affective science provides multiple exemplars where self-reporting of mental states is erroneous (Churchland, 2002; Gallagher, 2000; Goleman, 1996; Wegner, 2002). As noted above, like other schemas, self-schemas are only partial, and are subject to error. The point that a person's real interests and perceived interests are not necessarily the

---

[13] A discussion of authenticity ultimately leads to a discussion of what it is to be human, a point to which we return later.

[14] Over the course of the volume, it will become apparent that I am advocating an approach to authenticity that is not simply essentialist (e.g. less fear and more options) nor existentialist (i.e. wholly relativistic), but which requires that we aim for as comprehensive a knowledge of human beings and of particular individuals as possible (i.e. a humanistic and non-reductionistic naturalism).

same has been made since ancient times, and has been emphasized by a broad range of more recent thinkers (Bhaskar, 1979, 1986; Giddens, 1984; Thompson, 1984; Williams, 1985). As Socrates noted, "No physician, in so far as he is a physician knows himself" (Plato, 1997). Or as both Freud and Merleau-Ponty have pointed out more generally, consciousness is not completely transparent to itself. Indeed, a range of complex psychological and clinical phenomena, including self-deception, intra-personal conflict, and akrasia, may require concepts of the self that emphasize its fractured, non-conscious, and malleable nature (Radden, 1996).[15]

One way of understanding Abigail's case may be in terms of a disjunction between "disease" and "illness" (Frank, 1979; Kleinman, 1988; Stein, 1993).[16] "Disease" refers to structures and mechanisms that are altered by the pathology, while "illness" refers to the subjective expression and experience of the pathology. This is particularly useful in the clinic, where the clinician is required to negotiate with the patient about theories and values. When the clinician views the phenomena (e.g. social anxiety) as a disorder (e.g. SAD), and the patient disagrees (viewing her experience as normal temperament), then the clinician may usefully explore the patient's understanding, and try to come to a shared treatment plan. It should be noted that this framework does not assume that the patient's view is incommensurable with, or as valid as, the clinician's; rather there is an awareness of the importance of the clinician–patient relationship, and of setting reasonable goals that are able to incorporate scientific explanation as well as empathic understanding of patients' perspectives.

---

[15] As Johnson (1993) succinctly puts it

In a sense, we grope around for our identity, which is never a fixed or finished thing. It changes over time, while preserving some degree of continuity with our previous identities. That is why we can always be surprised by discovering new things about who we are, why we do what we do, and how others see us.

[16] Kleinman's view is perhaps partly related to, but also rather different from, the approaches taken by (1) Boorse (1975), where he argues that disease can be defined factually, whereas illness adds an evaluative component, and (2) Fulford (1989), where he argues that disease can be understood as a failure of function (in a part of a person), but illness is best understood as action failure (of the person).

5

Explanatory questions about psychotropics

In this chapter we cover a series of questions about explanations that are relevant to understanding philosophical issues in psychopharmacology. We have already begun to develop a particular contrast in philosophical discussion of explanations – the classical vs. critical approaches. The classical approach takes the view that it is possible to generate systematic generalizations or covering laws that describe the facts of the world (e.g. of the brain), and their relationships. The critical approach argues that human phenomena require a different kind of knowledge, one that is based on subjective understanding (e.g. of agents and their minds). The synthetic position taken here says that our brain-minds engage in various kinds of activity – both physical and social – are able to develop maps which provide explanations of the natural and human world, and can reasonably (cognitive-affectively) debate these maps and attempt to come up with ones that have greater explanatory power. Such explanatory power lies in understanding structures and their mechanisms (Bhaskar, 1978) and functions (Bolton & Hill, 1996).

In the next section this schema is used to discuss in turn how pharmacotherapy and psychotherapy work (which entails some discussion of brain-mind and nature–nurture relations), how placebo and nocebo effects occur (which leads to some discussion of symbolic grounding, and of the unconscious), and how evolutionary theory impacts on our understanding of cognitive-affective processes including those involved in the response to psychotropics and substances (which then involves some discussion of the constructs of function and dysfunction). As before, this schema of different approaches to explanation is an oversimplification, and as before rather than directly debating the contrasting views, we will put forward a conceptual position that is based in part on data from the cognitive-affective sciences.[1]

Psychotropics vs. psychotherapy – explaining brain-mind / nature–nuture

(A) Fabian Fanchetti came into the hospital complaining of obsessions and compulsions. He spent hours each day washing and cleaning, in order to make sure that he and his clothes were completely dirt-free. He put this down to growing up in a home where he's been taught that "cleanliness was next to godliness". Nevertheless, he knew that this behaviour was excessive, wanted to stop, but couldn't. He agreed to take part in a research project on obsessive–compulsive disorder (OCD), comparing the effects of medication and behavioural therapy on brain imaging. He was randomized to the medication arm, with a medication called clomipramine, and did well, experiencing a marked decrease in his symptoms. At first he found himself simply paying less attention to dirt, and feeling less anxious when he did not wash. By the end of the trial he felt that his prior behaviours had wasted years of his time, but that he was now free to live his life more fully. He learned that prior to treatment he had had increased activity in an area of the brain called the striatum, and that after treatment there had been a decrease in this activity. Furthermore, this same normalization of activity was also seen in subjects in the behavioural therapy arm of the study.

---

[1] In the concluding chapter I will discuss this methodology in more detail, addressing the relationship between philosophical and scientific approaches. An immediate objection to the approach here is to ask whether the selection of cognitive-affective data is biased to fit the conceptual position being defended ("cherry-picking"). While I accept that understanding of scientific data is theory-driven, I would argue that science does make progress, and that the science chosen here is the best available. Furthermore, only particularly sophisticated philosophical arguments will be able to underlabour for such science. Finally, in those cases where there is an absence of relevant cognitive-affective data, conceptual debates may be particularly difficult to resolve.

(B) *Gimoto Gasumatsu is a young woman who reported a history of repeated sexual abuse by her stepfather during childhood. As an adult she suffered from intrusive re-experiencing symptoms and difficulties in interpersonal relationships; she had difficulty in trusting people, and was often irritable with men. She agreed to take part in a research project on posttraumatic stress disorder (PTSD), assessing the size of the hippocampus. It turned out that the volume of her hippocampus was considerably smaller than those found in a healthy control group. As part of the study she received a trial of an SSRI; after treatment, she experienced a decrease in symptoms, and the volume of her hippocampus was noted to increase. At first she found that she was more comfortable in interpersonal situations involving men; she had an increased threshold for responding to comments with irritability. By the end of the trial, she also experienced fewer flashbacks to her past; she found herself "letting go" of her memory of and anger towards her stepfather. She continued on her pharmacotherapy for several months after the trial, and found that she was interested in establishing relationships with a new kind of man; whereas she had always been attracted to men who were aloof and interested only in non-committed sex, she now found herself wanting a closer relationship with a man who was interested in a more loving and longer-lasting relationship.*

How does pharmacotherapy work? How does psychotherapy work? Should there be different ways of understanding these two very different kinds of psychiatric intervention? These questions about the treatment of psychiatric disorders also raise the issue of how best to understand the origins of psychopathology – are psychiatric symptoms best understood in terms of underlying lawful associations (e.g. between neuronal or genetic abnormalities and particular behaviours), or as an understandable and intentional response (e.g. to a specific environmental context)? Such questions have been explored since ancient times (Simon, 1978), and they remain key for modern psychiatry and clinical psychopharmacology.[2]

---

[2] In the seventeenth century, Rousseau and Locke argued, respectively, that behavioural development was determined by unseen factors, or by the environment.

As outlined earlier, contrasting philosophical positions to science and to the mind underpin contrasting clinical approaches.[3] These clinical approaches emphasize different explanations, and, correspondingly, different treatments. Thus, a classical clinical position views psychopathology as a brain disorder, emphasizes associations between abnormal circuitry or genes and psychiatric symptoms, and is likely to suggest pharmacotherapy and behavioural therapy as treatment. In contrast, a critical clinical position, based on a view that psychopathology is an understandable response to the relevant context, typically focuses on the importance of meaning in both pathogenesis and psychotherapy.

A classical perspective may have some difficulty in accounting for the complex clinical cases described above. In particular, a reductionist view that focuses solely on the importance of basic physical laws in covering the data of the world, and which ignores emergent psychosocial mechanisms and functions, cannot easily describe how psychological trauma or psychotherapy leads to changes in neuronal function. As noted earlier, there has been a view that axis I disorders are best treated with medication, while axis II disorders are best treated with psychotherapy. However, increasingly there is evidence that genetic and environmental factors and nature–nurture interactions contribute to a range of psychopathology, and that both pharmacotherapy and psychotherapy are useful for a range of psychiatric symptoms.

A more sophisticated functionalist approach conceptualizes the mind in computational terms (Fodor, 1975; Putnam, 1967). Nevertheless, this position has not been employed successfully in the clinical arena either,

---

[3] A large philosophical literature focuses specifically on the so-called "mind–body problem", and a number of authors have examined these debates from the perspective of psychiatry (Goodman, 1991; Kendler, 2001; van Staden, 2006). Churchland (2002) comments, however, that there is only a mind–body "problem" if one accepts that the mind is non-physical and the body is physical, and certainly there are ongoing advances in detailing the psychobiology of complex brain-mind phenomena (Crick & Koch, 2003; Edelman, 2003). Still, there is the "hard problem" of how neurobiology produces consciousness (Chalmers, 1995). For others, however, explaining how mental states and conscious qualia emerge from the brain is in principle unsolvable, given our limited cognitive abilities (McGinn, 1989) (a position that has been called mysterian). Here we are primarily addressing a somewhat different, albeit related, set of questions about clinical phenomena and their explanation.

and ordinarily it pays little attention to the phylogenetic and ontogenetic origins of particular states of the brain-mind. Any idea that pharma-cotherapy acts on the hardware of the brain, while psychotherapy acts on the software, seems inadequate; after all, there is no distinction in the nervous system that corresponds to the division between hardware and software (Churchland, 2002). Indeed, a functionalist position that the brain substrate of mental states is essentially unimportant seems to harken back to the Cartesian division between the physicality of the body and the incorporality of the mental.

A critical perspective also has difficulty in accounting for the kinds of clinical cases described above. This approach has tended to be sceptical about whether psychotropics are in fact effective, or has viewed them as chemical straitjackets – simply exerting control in a different, per-haps more powerful way, than older physical methods of restraint and seclusion. The emphasis of this approach on the meaningfulness of psy-chiatric symptoms means that while it can readily view PTSD as a nor-mal response to an abnormal event (Small, 1984; Young, 1995), it may have difficulty in assimilating the contemporary view that this condi-tion is characterized by abnormalities in psychobiological mechanisms such as decreased hippocampal volume (Rauch *et al.*, 1998; Yehuda & McFarlane, 1995). Similarly, the critical approach has tended to view only meaning-oriented therapies as useful and worthwhile (Ingleby, 1981; Sedgwick, 1982).

However, critical perspective has perhaps been useful in pointing out how classically influenced approaches to pharmacotherapy and psychotherapy are incomplete. For example, there is a strong argu-ment that psychoanalytic psychotherapy relies on an outdated meta-psychology (emphasizing psychic energy), and that its recommended interventions are not evidence-based (Grünbaum, 1985; Stein, 1992). Further, there is now wide consensus that behaviourist models of the mind are necessarily incomplete (Gardner, 1985). And despite the evi-dence base for cognitive therapy, the hypothesis that distorted cognition leads to pathological emotions seems open to criticism. First, it appar-ently ignores a range of evidence that biological factors are crucial in the pathogenesis of psychiatric disorder. Second, it seems in conflict with current understandings of the way in which the brain-mind works; as discussed in detail earlier, we increasingly realize that cognition and affect are not neatly divorcible psychological faculties.

What do the data from cognitive-affective science say? Cognitive-affective science has investigated genetic and environmental mechanisms as well as the mechanisms altered by psychotropics and psychotherapy. Most modern psychotropics work by altering neuro-transmission in monoaminergic neurons that spread diffusely through the brain, and which therefore mediate a range of cognitive and affective processes. Some neuronal circuits may be particularly relevant to psychotherapy; prefrontal circuits, for example, play an important role in mediating extinction of fear, and may therefore also be altered by cognitive-behavioural interventions that reduce anxiety. Indeed, there is growing evidence that effective pharmacotherapies and psychotherapies are both able to normalize activity in specific neuronal circuits that mediate particular psychiatric symptoms (Baxter *et al.*, 1992; Furmark *et al.*, 2002; Paquetta *et al.*, 2003; Roffman *et al.*, 2005; Straube *et al.*, 2006).

Such work depends upon, and informs, an increasingly sophisticated understanding of the brain-mind. In the past, our maps of the brain-mind have been relatively crude; for example, a particularly common mapping has been of Mind as Container (Lakoff & Johnson, 1999). Freud, modern therapists, and lay people, are all able to talk about how "The painful thought has been pushed out of your mind". But modern cognitive-affective science is able to provide more detail on how particular neurocircuitry mediates cognitive-affective processes. Thus, we have moved from the nineteenth-century notions of energy flow through the brain, to early twentieth-century concepts of a "body schema", to more recent theories about how cognition (Maravita *et al.*, 2003) and affect (Damasio, 1996) are embodied in the brain-mind. This work should in turn lead to correspondingly sophisticated views on how to bring about changes in cognitive-affective processes.

Indeed, cognitive-affective science has been able to investigate the cognitive-affective characteristics of and alterations in particular neuronal circuits using a range of methods. Circuits can be explored bottom-up (i.e. their neurogenetics and neurochemistry can be delineated in detail) or top-down (i.e. their activation by particular psychological factors or within particular social environments can be investigated). This allows integrative explanations that include both low-level and high-level mechanisms and phenomena. This kind of approach is consistent with a non-reductionistic perspective on the relationship between different scientific disciplines, one that emphasizes the emergence of mental structures, mechanisms, and functions from the brain. Similarly, it allows an integration of cognitive-affective psychology with neuroscience (Churchland, 2002; Varela *et al.*, 1991), a joining of meaning with mechanism (Bhaskar, 1978; Bolton, 2004; Bolton & Hill, 1996; Schwartz & Wiggins, 1986), and an understanding of how nature and nurture interact to form the brain-mind (Dowling, 2004; Pinker, 2004; Ridley, 2003; Wexler, 2006) and its disorders (Caspi & Moffitt, 2006; Kendler, 2006).[4]

In discussing cognitive-affective science data in earlier parts of the volume, the discussion was divided into data from cognitive psychology, artificial intelligence, linguistics, neuroscience, developmental and evolutionary science, and philosophy. With advances in our maps of the brain-mind, and the use of multiple theories and methods to explore the mechanisms of pathogenesis and treatment, explanations of phenomena such as pharmacotherapy and psychotherapy increasingly cut across these disciplines. Work on changes in brain imaging induced by pharmacotherapy and psychotherapy, for example, requires incorporation of psychological and biological constructs, and may be modelled using neural networks. Work in developmental science similarly is shedding increasing light on the precise nature of interactions between gene and environment, and on understanding the development of the brain-mind in its particular context, while work on evolutionary theory of the brain-mind also aims to be grounded in biological and ecological mechanisms (Panksepp & Panksepp, 2000). Philosophical work has created the space to move beyond explanations of the brain-mind that rely solely on physical or intentional constructs, and that emphasize rather how meaning is encoded in the brain-mind, and grounded in

---

[4] This kind of view therefore avoids what has been termed "geneticization" (Lippman, 1992), which can be understood as a particularly reductionistic approach within a classical view of medicine.

the interaction of people with their contexts (Bhaskar, 1978; Bolton, 2004; Bolton & Hill, 1996).[5]

Returning to the cases described above, it seems overly simplistic, for example, to say that the serotonergic antidepressant, clomipramine, is effective in a particular disorder, such as OCD, because this disorder is characterized by a pathological serotonin system (van Praag, 2000). Serotonergic circuits are likely to play a role in mediating a broad range of normal behaviours and pathological symptoms; this is consistent with the fact that these neurons branch widely through the brain, and that they appear to have a general modulatory role. Thus, rather than mediating any particular behaviour, clomipramine may act to change the firing setpoint for a large number of neurons, involved in a wide variety of functions. By changing the activity of striatal and related circuits, which are involved in cognitive-affective processes such as set-switching and control of procedural strategies, clomipramine reduces obsessions and compulsions in OCD, but also improves symptoms in other kinds of disorders. (From a philosophical perspective, clomipramine has an intentional component in that it alters the serotonergic system, but a non-intentional causal effect in relation to cognitive-affective processes and psychopathology (Bolton & Hill, 1996).)

Similarly, it is unlikely that we can develop an explanation of behavioural exposure during psychotherapy which does not involve brain. OCD, for example, is characterized by increased activity in the cortico–striatal–thalamic–cortical (CSTC) circuits involved in

[5] As noted earlier, a non-reductionistic realist approach to complex phenomena makes space for a range of theories and methods. Nevertheless, an ontological gap (Kriel, 2000) between different levels of reality, or an explanatory gap (Levine, 1983) in our accounts of their relationship, may be noted. Ghaemi (2003) contrasts an eclectic and pragmatic biopsychosocial approach (in which any explanation goes), with an integrationist approach (in which there is an attempt to focus on integrative explanations), and a pluralist approach (in which certain accounts are viewed as more valid in particular circumstances). The term "psychobiological" emphasizes the increasing integration of the biological and the psychological, and the idea that behaviour has to be understood both in terms of its overall meaning and underlying mechanism. As Merleau-Ponty notes, there are no explanations without comprehension (Merleau-Ponty, 1962). At the same time, a view which emphasizes that several causal mechanisms are involved in any disorder, and that some models are more valid than others for particular cases, is consistent with the approach taken throughout this volume. Mitchell (2003) has proposed the persuasive term "integrative pluralism".

particular cognitive-affective functions (such as set-switching and control of procedural strategies). Both clomipramine and behavioural therapy are able to decrease activity in these circuits (Baxter *et al.*, 1992). A similar change may well be brought about by particular kinds of cognitive therapy. Cognitive-affective processes are embodied in the brain, and can be changed by the causal effects of both non-intentional (psychotropic) and intentional (psychotherapeutic) interventions (Bolton & Hill, 1996). (From a philosophical perspective, in order to explain fully how an intervention that focuses primarily on meaning (psychotherapy) exerts its effects, we need to understand the underlying brain-mind mechanisms that underpin that meaning (Bhaskar, 1979).)

Although the kinds of explanations offered here to explain clinical cases may seem obvious enough, this approach has significant implications for a number of debates in philosophy of psychology and of cognitive science (Clark, 2001; Goldman, 1993b; Greenwood, 1991; Ramsay *et al.*, 1991). The functionalist view that has been so popular in contemporary cognitive science divorces the software and hardware of the mind; the brain-mind is conceptualized in terms of its functional states. In this volume we do not address these debates directly; rather, the emphasis is on the conceptual point that such a model simply does not allow for sufficiently powerful explanations of clinical phenomena. A functionalist explanation of the efficacy of medication and of psychotherapy would necessarily be in terms of using psychotherapy to change the software, and medication to change the hardware of the mind. But the reality is clearly more complex than this, with clinical research documenting the effects of psychotherapy on brain, and the effects of psychotropics on cognitive-affective processes. Thus, the hardware–software distinction simply fails to describe adequately the brain-mind (Churchland, 2002; Lakoff & Johnson, 1999), and the way in which it mediates psychiatric pathology and intervention. Instead, we need a conceptual approach that recognizes the unique "wetware" that underpins the embodied brain-mind and its interaction with the world.

Such a conceptual approach may also be able to go beyond the debate in cognitive science between symbolic cognitivists and situated cognitivists (Norman, 1993). Symbolic cognitivists take a position reminiscent of the classical perspective, arguing that cognitive processing essentially involves the manipulation of symbols, which are independent of their physical instantiation. Situated cognitivists, on the other hand, hold that cognitive processes necessarily take place within a particular interactive social context, emphasize concepts such as ecology (Neisser, 1976) and affordances (Gibson, 1977) to emphasize the environment and the properties of things in the environment that are relevant to the kinds of interactions that people have with them, and prefer computational models such as neural networks or robotic agents that operate within particular environments. Some of the arguments against symbolic cognitivism are reminiscent of the critical position; Searle, for example, emphasizes the importance of human intentionality, arguing that this simply cannot be captured by formal cognitivist models (Searle, 1983, 2006).[6] From the synthetic or integrative perspective taken here, however, a cognitivist position can be developed that emphasizes the embodiment of mind in sensorimotor-affective circuits, with the grounding of cognitive-affective maps in direct interactions with the physical and social world (Bolton & Hill, 1996; Clark, 1997; Harnad, 1990).

Placebo vs. nocebo – explaining symbol grounding/ the unconscious

Harold Hannemeyer made an appointment at his local psychiatric hospital outpatient clinic. He had always been a tidy and hygienic person, but over the last few years his cleaning routine had gotten out of control. He spent several hours a day washing his hands and cleaning his apartment, in order to make sure there were no germs. He realized that this was excessive, but felt too embarrassed to discuss it with anyone. However, things were now at the point where he was beginning to feel demoralized and depressed by how much time he wasted, and by how little time he had to do anything productive. At the clinic he was told about a research trial of a new medication that might be helpful for people with obsessive–compulsive

---

[6] Searle ignores the crucial point that symbols have meaning because they are linked to sensorimotor capacities and to interaction with the environment (Bolton & Hill, 1996).

disorder (OCD). He agreed to take part, and within a few months was doing
much better. At the end of the trial he elected to continue with the same
medication, now given open-label. Within a day, he experienced intense
nausea, and could no longer continue with the medication. It turned out
he had been on placebo all along.[7]

Randomized clinical trials (RCTs) are the gold standard of evidence-based medicine (Leber, 2000; Sackett *et al.*, 1996), despite their limitations (Cartwright, 2007). The use of a placebo control is the best available methodology for differentiating the specific therapeutic effects and adverse events of a new medication from the non-specific placebo and nocebo effects of an inert substance. In this classical position, a placebo tablet represents "noise": it is a non-specific effect that must be subtracted from the specific effects of medication, so that the signal demonstrating efficacy can be seen more clearly (Harrington, 1999; Shapiro & Shapiro, 2001). This may contribute to explaining why mechanisms underlying placebo effects have not been particularly well explored, despite the fact that placebo is the most effective of all medical interventions (at least in terms of its breadth of therapeutic activity; Guess *et al.*, 2002; White *et al.*, 1985).

For the critical position, controlled clinical trials are not so much the foundation of medical science, but part of a fallible system that has no absolute foundations (Cartwright, 2007). Furthermore, placebo effects underline that psychiatric disorders are ultimately social in nature. If OCD were really a neurological disorder, like Parkinson's disorder, there would be less-robust placebo effects in OCD clinical trials. The meaningfulness of a diagnostic label and a therapeutic relationship is sufficiently powerful that patients with psychiatric disorders can respond to medication even when it is inert. Indeed, a great deal has been written about the meaning of the placebo (Brody, 1980; Moerman, 2002). As Brody (2000) states, when an encounter with a healer changes the meaning of the illness experience in a positive direction, then there is more likely to be a placebo response. This is particularly likely when the individual receives a meaningful explanation, when he/she feels care

---

[7] There is a small bioethics literature on what to do in this situation (Di Blasi *et al.*, 2002).

and concern, and when there is an enhanced sense of mastery or control over the illness.

What does cognitive-affective science say? We can begin by noting that although evidence-based medicine is sometimes caricatured in classical terms, good evidence-based practice integrates research evidence with both clinical expertise and patient values (Sackett *et al.*, 1996; Stein *et al.*, 2005). Further, although it is important to separate placebo effects from measurement artefacts (Hrobjartsson & Gotzsche, 2001; McDonald *et al.*, 1983), most agree that a placebo response is present in many medical and psychiatric disorders, and advances in neurochemistry and functional imaging have helped elucidate the underlying psychobiology (Stein & Mayberg, 2005). Thus, in Parkinson's disorder placebo responders demonstrate increased dopamine release, consistent with basic work showing such release during reward anticipation (de la Fuente-Fernandez *et al.*, 2001; de la Fuente-Fernández & Stoessl, 2004). Work on depressed patients who respond to placebo shows specific activation/deactivation patterns in cortical–limbic circuits on functional brain imaging consistent with a role for expectancy effects (Leuchter *et al.*, 2002; Mayberg *et al.*, 2002). In investigating response to an active psychotropic, we therefore need to explore both non-intentional processes (e.g. the neurotransmitter effects of the psychotropic: conditioning effects) and intentional processes (e.g. cognitive-affective processing focused on the value of being prescribed a psychotropic: expectancy effects; Bolton & Hill, 1996).

Indeed, placebo and nocebo responses can ultimately be understood using the same type of schema outlined earlier for understanding the mechanism of action of pharmacotherapy and of psychotherapy. First, the underlying neurocircuitry and its associated cognitive-affective functions are delineated. Second, bottom-up (neurogenetics, neurochemistry, etc.) and top-down (psychological, social, etc.) investigations are undertaken. The bottom-up approach indicates that in Parkinson's disease the dopamine system plays a role in mediating placebo effects, while in depression cortico-limbic circuits are important. One could predict (if not yet demonstrate) that psychological and social factors important in expectancy effects (Brody, 2000) are ultimately also able to alter the relevant neurochemistry and neurocircuitry. A different constellation of psychobiological and psychosocial factors may, however, result in a nocebo effect. Furthermore, an evolutionary perspective may suggest that expectancies in social situations reflect our evolved cognitive abilities, and that capacity to have expectancies in therapeutic contexts in particular may have an evolutionary advantage (Bendesky & Sonabend, 2005; Evans, 2003; Humphrey, 2002).

A detailed consideration of the ethics of using placebo in randomized controlled trials is beyond the scope of the current volume. Nevertheless, it is notable that a philosophical position has gradually emerged which emphasizes the complexity of such decisions (Emanuel & Miller, 2001). Thus, a particular placebo-controlled design which is less acceptable in one context (where the active medication is already known to be effective, for example) may be more acceptable in another (where it may still be necessary to demonstrate the cost-efficacy of the active medication, for example). Such a view goes beyond a classical view of placebo as merely noise and also beyond a critical view that is entirely sceptical of the value of randomized placebo-controlled clinical trials, and is consistent with a view of placebo and nocebo responses as complex brain-mind phenomena that are mediated by psychobiological mechanisms and that take place within particular psychosocial contexts.

Indeed, the question arises of the implications of our accounts of placebo and nocebo responses for models of the brain-mind. They demand a model that is not merely symbolic or functional, but that at the same time can ground meaning in psychobiological mechanisms. One interesting philosophical answer to the question of how symbols are grounded so that they have meaning has been put forward by Harnad, who describes an elegant variant of the Turing Test, the Total Turing Test (TTT; Harnad, 1989). In addition to simulation of pen-pal (symbolic) interactions, passing the TTT demands simulation of "robotic capacity" – all of our sensorimotor capacity to discriminate, recognize, identify, manipulate, and describe the world we live in. Harnard argues that a system is grounded only when it has the symbolic and robotic capacity to pass the TTT test in a coherent way; that is, when its symbolic capacity is grounded in its robotic capacity (so that cognition is embodied).

A machine that responded to particular psychotropic agents that also work in humans would be extremely similar to humans, to the point that it would likely be more of a phenocopy than a model. More interesting, perhaps, would be a machine that did not necessarily respond to pharmaceuticals, but that did respond to placebos. Indeed, it might be suggested that any machine that is sufficiently complex to pass the TTT would necessarily respond to placebos. It would not simply be a cognitive processing machine, but would also be an affect processing machine. Such a machine would have sufficiently complex grounded symbolic capacity, and sufficiently complex interactions, that it would find the administration of placebos meaningful. This could be called the placebo Turing test (PTT).

The placebo response also raises the question of how best to conceptualize the unconscious. The person who experiences a response to placebo remains unaware of how factors such as the therapeutic relationship, and changes in the meaning of the illness experience, result in a therapeutic response. Of course, a lack of awareness by owners of brain-minds of how brain-mind structures and mechanisms lead to thoughts, feelings, and behaviours, is the rule. Thus, both psychoanalysis and cognitive science agree that the majority of mental processing takes place outside of awareness. However, where Freud's concept of the unconscious relied on nineteenth-century concepts of energy, cognitive science has developed a rather different approach to the unconscious, emphasizing the contrast between implicit and explicit cognitive and affective processes (Kihlstrom, 1987; Stein, 1997).

There are many within the classical tradition who have been sceptical of the notion that psychoanalysis is a science (Clark & Wright, 1988; Grünbaum, 1985; Hook, 1959; Popper, 1974; Wollheim & Hopkins, 1982). Wittgenstein (1982) suggested that Freud had muddled causes with reasons. As briefly noted above, the objective and ahistorical emphasis of much classical thinking conflicts with psychodynamic theory's embrace of the subjective and of the historic. On the other hand, a number of authors in the psychodynamic tradition have argued that psychoanalysis has the structure of other sciences, and that its laws cover unconscious phenomena. There are strands within this tradition that emphasize the energetics underlying mental phenomena

(Bilder & LeFever, 1998; Ellenberger, 1970), or more recently, the way in which the unconscious can be re-conceptualized in terms of symbolic representations (Bowers & Meichenbaum, 1984; Erdelyi, 1985) or brain-mind embodiment (Solms & Turnbull, 2003; Zacharacopoulou, 2006).

Similarly, within the critical tradition, psychoanalysis has had severe critics. For much of the twentieth century, psychoanalysis was the predominant paradigm of American psychiatry, and was therefore open to accusations of being a non-progressive means of social control. On the other hand, a number of authors in the psychodynamic tradition have argued that psychoanalysis is a human science, and that its particular approach to narrative and interpretation provides unique insights. As noted earlier, some have conceptualized psychotherapy in terms of narrative text, have emphasized the intersubjective aspects of analytic phenomena such as the transference, or have focused on the discursive nature of the unconscious (Habermas, 1971; Klein, 1976; Mitchell, 1988; Ricoeur, 1970, 1981; Schafer, 1976).

From the perspective of cognitive-affective science, the unconscious cognitive-affective processes that mediate placebo and nocebo responses, as well as a range of other complex brain-mind phenomena, can be understood by exploring their underlying neuronal circuitry and molecular mechanisms. Once again, the relevant structures and mechanisms can be investigated empirically using both bottom-up (neurogenetics, neurochemistry, etc.) and top-down (psychological, social, etc.) methodologies. Psychodynamic constructs and theories may change considerably during this process of investigation, but a cognitive-affective science of the unconscious with a good deal of explanatory power may emerge (Stein *et al.*, 2006).[8] Thus, while a Cartesian approach may have allowed objectification of the body, in order to develop appropriately complex explanations of psychiatric phenomena, and their underlying (unconscious) cognitive-affective processes, a

---

[8] Similar considerations may well apply to conscious processes and free will (Armstrong & Malcolm, 1984; Block *et al.*, 1997; Chalmers, 1995; Churchland, 1995; Dennett, 1991, 2003; Dilman, 1999; Humphrey, 1999; Kane, 2001; Libet *et al.*, 1999; Lloyd, 2004; Marijuán, 2001; Searle, 2006; Spence *et al.*, 2002; Walter, 2001; Watson, 2003; Wegner, 2002), but these topics go beyond our focus here.

detailed understanding of the way in which these processes are grounded in the brain-mind is necessary (Leder, 1984).[9]

This kind of understanding of the placebo process is not merely theoretical, but may have important clinical implications. As noted earlier, a good physician needs to understand not only disease, but also illness (the meaning of the disorder). On the one hand, it is important to avoid objectification of the patient (ignoring the particular circumstances and context of symptoms); on the other hand, it is important not to overlook the diagnosis of medical conditions and the value of psychotropic agents in patients who present with apparently meaningful behavioural symptoms. A model of the brain-mind that simultaneously provides explanations of mechanism and meaning, of symbols and their grounding, of context and its brain-mind embodiment, is therefore key for good medical practice, including good psychopharmacology. Before going on to consider the notion of good pharmacotherapy in more detail in the next chapter, we consider distal (evolutionary) explanations of psychiatric disorders and treatments.

Evolutionary psychopharmacology – explaining function/dysfunction

He who understands baboon would do more towards metaphysics than Locke (Darwin, 1838)

Before entering the trial of clomipramine versus behavioural therapy, Fabian had been convinced that his washing obsessions and compulsions were the consequence of his family environment. When he was a child, the importance of cleanliness had always been emphasized. He also suspected that family conflict played a role – he always felt pulled in one way by his father, and in another by his mother, and this seemed to relate to his perpetual uncertainty about things. However, as he learned more about clomipramine, and its effects in people with OCD, he changed his

[9] Merleau-Ponty (1942) helped lay the path for such a strategy by arguing that Freud's energic metaphors needed to be replaced by structural metaphors. He argued that "structure" is the philosophical truth of naturalism and realism.

explanatory model. He was particularly interested to learn from his doctor that clomipramine is effective in dogs with excessive grooming behaviour; so-called acral lick dermatitis. He decided that just as acral lick dermatitis represents excessive activation of grooming in canines, so OCD represents a kind of false alarm in humans. This notion was instrumental in his decision to continue medication after the end of the trial.

Insofar as the classical perspective downplays the social and cultural context of science, it has often been ahistorical in its approach. Perhaps this helps to explain why in medicine and psychiatry the focus has been so much on the proximal factors involved in disease, with relatively little attention paid to its distal evolutionary origins (MacLean, 1985; Nesse & Williams, 1994). Similarly, it may help explain why the Freudian emphasis on the origins of mental function and psychopathology in childhood experience has been so negatively received by philosophers (Grünbaum, 1985). Less speculatively, it is notable that early conceptual analyses criticized biology for not following sufficiently well in the footsteps of physics (Mayr, 1988; Ruse, 1989). With the rapid advances in biological science, and a firm basis in evolutionary explanations, a rich conceptual basis for biology has developed (Grene & Depew, 2004; Hull & Ruse, 2007; Mayr, 1988; Ruse, 1989), and there has been growing scientific interest in evolutionary approaches in medicine and psychiatry.

The critical perspective has by and large placed a great deal of emphasis on social and cultural context. Freud, for example, has been commended by many in the critical camp, not as a scientist, but as a deep thinker who addresses the meaningfulness of mental phenomena (Ricoeur, 1970). Furthermore, Mayr (1988) has argued that the switch from classical essentialist thinking to population thinking is what made the theory of evolution possible; the genotype is shaped by the context of all its preceding ancestors, and there is no corresponding kind of distal explanation in the physical sciences. Nevertheless, for the critical thinker, context is typically conceptualized in terms of human society and culture, rather than in evolutionary terms. Given the importance of meaning and language for the critical perspective, there is a clear division between animal and human minds, a scepticism about the implications of evolutionary theory for psychology, and an acute awareness that social practices need not be selected for by evolution. Such views have been emphasized by more critical philosophers of biology (Kitcher, 1985; Levins & Lewontin, 1985; Midgley, 1978; Rose, 1998b; Rose & Rose, 2000; Rose & The Dialectics of Biology Group, 1982; Ruse, 1979).

What does cognitive-affective science say? Cognitive-affective science is keenly aware of biological continuities between animals and humans, and describing the evolution of structures and mechanisms across species is of crucial interest. Evolutionary psychology has increasingly become incorporated as one of the sub-disciplines of cognitive science (Buss, 2005; Cosmides & Tooby, 2003; Wright, 1995), responsible for augmenting proximate psychobiological explanations with distal evolutionary ones. The brain-mind must be understood as an evolutionary product, an adaptation that allows the organism to function more effectively in its particular niche (Duchaine *et al.*, 2001). Nevertheless, there are many questions that remain unresolved when this framework is applied to psychopathology. For this volume an immediate question is whether evolutionary psychology provides a useful framework for thinking about, and providing explanations of, psychiatric disorders and their pharmacotherapy.

An important goal for the field of evolutionary psychology is the development of models of homeostatic (in-balance) and allostatic (out-of-balance) cognitive-affective processes that can be investigated across species. If the brain-mind mechanisms underlying repetitive behaviours have evolved gradually over time, for example, then the study of habits in rodents may turn out to involve homologous psychobiological structures and functions that are involved in normal repetitive behaviour and abnormal obsessive–compulsive behaviours in humans. Indeed, it is quite remarkable that excessive canine grooming responds to the same psychotropic medication that works for OCD symptoms, suggesting that similar neurocircuitry mediates both phenomena (Rapoport *et al.*, 1992).

Similarly, an evolutionary perspective helps to explain why a handful of psychotropics have such powerful effects across behaviours and across species (Stein, 1998, 2006). The power of these agents resides not so much in their own structure as in the effect that they may have on complex, evolved, endogenous neurocircuitry. This holds for both therapeutic drugs and abused substances (a category that, as noted earlier, overlaps; Nesse & Berridge, 1997). Cannabis works not like a hammer to disrupt the brain-mind, but rather via endogenous cannabinoid receptors, finely tuned by evolution, on which the drug acts to alter cognitive-affective processes. Analogously, the famous and infamous SSRI, Prozac (or fluoxetine), works because it modulates a system that has survived across eons of evolutionary history in multiple species. Thus, both rodents and primates (including humans) get drunk on alcohol, and have increased motivation on antidepressants.

What are the implications, then, for this kind of evolutionary thinking for thinking about and explaining psychiatric disorder? One approach, consistent with a more classical emphasis on covering laws, is that disorders can be accounted for in terms of an evolutionary account of dysfunction. In this view, we can then differentiate between states of unhappiness, of demoralization, and of the disorder of depression, on the basis of whether an explanation involving dysfunction is relevant. Whereas unhappiness (Buss, 2000), and demoralization (Nesse, 2000) may have adaptive functions, there are cases of depression that are characterized by dysfunction. Indeed, several authors have tried to define disorder in evolutionary theoretical terms as a "biological disadvantage" (Scadding, 1967) or "design failure" (Wakefield, 1999a).

Consistent with a more critical perspective that emphasizes subjective and contextual understandings, however, it might be argued that evolutionary accounts may well provide an understanding of the origins and adaptiveness of behaviour, but this does not mean that they yield definitions of "function" or "dysfunction" in necessary and sufficient terms. A key question is whether evolutionary explanations are sufficient to differentiate the idea that the function of the heart is to pump blood from the argument that the sounds of the heart function to allow us to listen to it, and then whether we can differentiate disorder from normal variants (Hempel, 1965; Wakefield, 1999a). Critics of an essential approach would argue that biological and evolutionary explanations are too complex to yield classical conclusions of the form, "the function of the heart is to pump blood", "a heart disorder occurs when this function goes awry".

While it might be fair, for example, to begin with a first step of saying that the function of the heart is to pump blood, a range of other complicating considerations soon come in to play. For a particular elderly person, a certain cardiac output may be enough to live with good quality of life, but for a more robust individual, it may be considered crucial to have a much higher ventricular ejection. There might be a gene variant in the population which proves adaptive under some circumstances (e.g. increasing cardiac output early in life, which may allow superior athleticism and improve survival in certain contexts), but maladaptive in other circumstances (e.g. leading to vulnerability to earlier death, which may decrease life span and diminish survival in other contexts). Thus, while understanding genes and their variations may provide powerful explanations of medical phenomena, such knowledge may not provide a nosology entirely mapped to genes (Kendler, 2006). Similarly, although cognitive-affective science may usefully emphasize the value of evolutionary explanations, this may lead to an appreciation of human diversity rather than to a neat dichotomy between function and dysfunction (Troisi, 2005).

In a discussion relevant to the considerations here, Polyani (1958) suggested that we look for reasons for the way biological systems work, but that we emphasize instead the causes of their failure. In this view, evolutionary theory might be particularly useful in understanding the survival of normal psychobiological mechanisms, while other kinds of non-intentional explanations would be needed to explain pathology. However, as Bolton and Hill (1996) emphasize, breakdown can also result from intentional processes. In sickle cell anaemia, for example, the underlying responsible trait appears to be inherited because of its ability to confer protection against malaria.[10] In some cases of impulsive-aggression, the relevant genetic variant may survive because of the benefit conferred in resource-limited environments. Explanations

---

[10] This exemplar is also discussed by Boorse (1997) and by Wakefield (1999a), who argue that the existence of such an inherited problem is not a design failure. However, I think Wakefield fails to address adequately the point that variants (including extreme variants) are maintained in the population by selection pressure.

of medical disorder often entail an interplay between intentional and non-intentional causal processes.[11]

Wakefield's view of disorder as "harmful dysfunction" (1992a, 1993, 1995, 1997, 1999a, 1999b, 2001) potentially allows him to combine both objective and value-laden factors in defining disorder, while retaining a naturalistic approach to explanations (which focus on why humans are made like they are). It is therefore attractive in a number of ways, and appears to be an advance over earlier approaches to defining disease solely in terms of malfunction (Boorse, 1975). Nevertheless, he adheres rigorously to the logic of an essentialist approach to dysfunction. In response to a broad range of counter-examples of the kind noted above (Lilienfeld & Marino., 1995, 1999), he emphasizes the explanatory power of evolutionary accounts, and argues that such accounts differentiate disorders from non-disorders. When there is a conflict of evolutionary accounts of function with human practices and values, he downplays the latter (arguing, for example, that decreased cardiac output as one ages is not a dysfunction, having gene variants that are associated with high levels of trait aggression is not a disorder). This leads to a view in which many conditions that are currently viewed as disorders are defined as non-disorders (Bolton, 2000).

For example, Wakefield argues that social anxiety disorder should only be diagnosed when anxiety reaches debilitating levels in species expectable tasks (Wakefield *et al.*, 2005), and that current operational diagnostic criteria lead to overdiagnosis of such conditions (Spitzer & Wakefield, 1999).[12] Nevertheless, as alluded to earlier, there

---

[11] For detailed discussion of the philosophy of causal and non-causal (e.g., reason-based or folk psychology) theories of action, see Bhaskar (1979) on the human sciences in general, and Fulford and colleagues (2006) on psychiatry in particular. Similarly, psychotropics can perhaps work in an intentional or a non-intentional way (Bolton, personal communication). As noted earlier, serotonin reuptake inhibitors act on a finely tuned endogenous system, likely upregulating serotonergic responses to the environment. On the other hand, certain nootropics may act to enhance neuronal protection in general.

[12] Spitzer and Wakefield (1999) argue that the so-called "clinical significance criterion" in DSM-IV is conceptually weak, and may lead to overdiagnosis of psychiatric disorders. However, there is also the possibility that the clinical significance criterion leads to underestimation of psychiatric disorders in various populations (Coyne & Marcus, 2006; Jablensky, 2005).

is uncertainty about whether or not social anxiety disorder reflects a design failure, and there is a strong argument that many cases are associated with significant distress and impairment and deserve to be conceptualized as disorders (Campbell-Sills & Stein, 2005). Similarly, although it may be argued that in many cases excessive use of alcohol does not involve an underlying design failure, this condition can nevertheless be validly considered a disorder (i.e. alcoholism; Clark, 2007.)[13] Whereas Wakefield wants to revise the current nosology to omit such conditions, other evolutionary thinkers accept that evolutionary accounts of function and dysfunction diverge markedly from ordinary human standards of value (so that dysfunctions can be beneficial, while mechanisms that perform their evolved function can cause disturbing outcomes; Cosmides & Tooby, 1999) or emphasize that various phenomena (e.g. nausea during pregnancy, depression after a loss, impulsivity in certain social contexts) challenge the notion that disorders are essences distinctly separate from normal conditions (Nesse, 2001).

While Wakefield (1999b) wants "dysfunction" to serve as an essential natural kind that defines disorder, our view here would instead be that insofar as the concept of dysfunction provides an explanation that is similar to that used in the breakdown metaphor of disorder, it provides a useful shorthand for thinking about medical and psychiatric conditions and their explanations. Similarly, Lilienfeld and Marino note that at the heart of the prototype of disorder is an account that "there is something wrong with the body or mind that needs to be fixed" (Lilienfeld & Marino, 1999). The attempt, however, to explain the function (and corresponding dysfunction) of humans is one that goes back at least to Aristotle (Megone, 1998), and that remains an ongoing project (Berlin, 1980; Berry, 1986; Bhaskar, 1986; Blackford, 2006; Buller, 2005; Malik, 2000; Reynolds, 1976; Richards, 2000; Shotter, 1975). While it has been suggested that an emphasis on the human functions of reasoning

---

[13] The argument here is not necessarily only about psychiatric disorders. Wakefield (1999a) has argued that design/environment mismatch obesity should not be considered a disorder, and that cosmetic surgery cannot be conceptualized in terms of being used to treat a disorder. These points do not seem defensible.

capacity (Megone, 1998), or of moral sentiment (Schaffner, 1999), provide a useful basis for conceptualizing disorder, what counts as a good reason or a right moral are open to contestation. Indeed, the social frame into which one is born influences the way one understands and pursues such goals as surviving and flourishing (Johnson, 1993). Thus, to conceptualize and explain human nature and medical disorders in a comprehensive way, we have to go beyond a natural science perspective on the way the body and the brain work, to include also a consideration of human practices and values (Fulford, 2002; Thornton, 2002).[14]

In brief, the integrative conceptual approach taken here is that while scientific explanations, including evolutionary explanations, may not yield an essentialist or algorithmic solution to defining and understanding human nature or medical disorders, they are nevertheless useful in informing the relevant debate on concepts about and explanations of these phenomena. In a typical disorder, there may be little debate, as it is clear, from whichever perspective one adopts, that there is a "break-down", which is impairing, and that intervention can potentially reverse the breakdown and associated impairment. In the less typical case, however, explanations from natural science, social science, and evolutionary science may yield conflicting conclusions (a cognitive science study may indicate that impulsive traits are associated with impairment in decision-making, while an evolutionary study may note that impulsive traits are associated with increased achievement in particular contexts), and considerations that emphasize clinical utility (e.g. the use of a diagnosis to shape treatment decisions) may conflict with considerations that prioritize explanatory power (i.e. the use of a diagnosis to emphasize etiology; First *et al.*, 2004; Kendell & Jablensky, 2003; Kendler, 1990; Rounsaville *et al.*, 2002; Zachar & Kendler, 2007).

---

[14] There is an interesting debate between Wakefield (1999a) and Lilienfeld and Marino (1999) on whether dyslexia, amusia, etc., can be explained by an evolutionary analysis. I agree with Lilienfeld and Marino that there is no evolutionarily based reason for viewing these conditions, rather than say inability to cook, as disorders. However, I disagree with Lilienfeld and Marino, in that I think that classifying such conditions as disorders can be argued scientifically (and part of the reasoning might include an evolutionary analysis of brain functioning).

As suggested in the earlier chapter on the construct of clinical disorder, debate about how best to classify and conceptualize a condition should therefore include a reasoned, and continuously updated, consideration of our shared cognitive-affective maps of disorder, of our knowledge of the relevant medical (including evolutionary) science, and of the details of the specific clinical cases at hand.

The growing literature on evolutionary medicine is increasingly sophisticated, and so already provides a solid basis for an innovative and integrative approach to understanding disorder (Cosmides & Tooby, 1999; Mealey, 1997; Nesse, 2001). Nesse and Williams (1994) note that evolutionary explanations of pathology rely on constructs such as evolutionary trade-offs (different traits are adaptive in different environments), genome lag (evolved traits may be out of step with current environments), and historical constraints (how a trait has evolved may result in particular susceptibility to disease). They emphasize that many evolved defences (e.g. pain) and tendencies (e.g. impulsivity) may allow gene survival, but may harm our own lives.[15] In the extreme case, for example, where a gene variant results in early death, we can certainly agree that there is a disorder and harmful dysfunction. But in more atypical cases (e.g. many cases of social anxiety, alcoholism), there may be no harmful dysfunction (i.e. no design failure from an evolutionary perspective), but we may nevertheless reasonably agree that a disorder is present (e.g. given the accompanying clinical distress and negative impact).

Given the focus of this volume on cosmetic psychopharmacology, it may be useful to consider the quite subtle example of ageing (Caplan, 1981; Nesse & Williams, 1994; Post & Binstock, 2004). Is ageing best explained as a function (design) or dysfunction (design failure)? Or is it simply a condition of life (Davis, 2004; Rose, 2002)? It turns out that a species that is sexual and then ages has adaptive advantages compared with one that is not sexual and lives longer, so that from an evolutionary perspective ageing can be explained in functional terms.

---

[15] Wakefield (1999a) responds to these kinds of exemplars by saying that he wants to capture design failure rather than design/environment mismatch, for "that is how humans are designed". However, this does not seem a persuasive response – many adaptations can reasonably be judged to be disorders.

However, in progeria, a rare condition, there is premature ageing prior to procreation – in this prototypical instance, from an evolutionary perspective, this can be understood in terms of a design failure. Similarly, premature Alzheimer's disorder, with severe cognitive impairment in one's thirties or forties, can arguably be explained in terms of a design failure.

However, a few centuries ago, living into one's seventies would be considered remarkable, whereas nowadays conditions such as osteoarthritis, atherosclerosis, prostatism, as well as mild cognitive impairment, in one's seventies are all considered disorders even when they begin at this relatively late stage of life (Dekkers & Rikkert, 2007; Petersen *et al.*, 2001). Now these are arguably not best explained as design failures (given that the human body is designed to procreate long before senescence, rather than to have optimal functioning during senescence). Further, the benefits of anti-ageing interventions have often been exaggerated (Turner, 2004). So perhaps disorders associated with ageing are best viewed as atypical disorders. But they would seem to be disorders, none the less. Wakefield's necessary and sufficient criteria, and consequent explanations of medical phenomena, may hold for the prototypic centre (i.e. of the disorder progeria, and its explanation as a dysfunction) – as noted, his constructs overlap with the common "mechanical breakdown" metaphor of disorder – but they fail at the boundaries of disorder.

There may be a deeper problem with evolutionary psychology as a whole (perhaps reflecting an over-reliance on classical rule-based concepts). On the one hand, evolutionary psychology performs a valuable service, in emphasizing that not only proximal but also distal mechanisms must be considered in explanations (Nesse *et al.*, 1994). On the other hand, evolutionary psychologists sometimes appear to take a Platonic stance to the mind, hypothesizing such formal constructs as a "language module", or a "cheating module", without specifically exploring the underlying brain-mind mechanisms that would underpin these psychological faculties. It is open to debate, however, as to whether evolution psychology should rely, as it so often does, on notions of algorithmically defined (Dennett, 1995) behavioural modules (Churchland, 2002; Cosmides & Tooby, 2003; Panksepp & Panksepp, 2000).

The counter-argument (perhaps reflecting a critical perspective on mind and on contexts) is that during evolution there are changes in genes, and specific genes are likely to affect general aspects of cognitive-affective functioning, as well as gene–environment inter-actions, rather than rule-based behavioural modules. Thus, a sin-gle nucleotide polymorphism in a particular gene may have multi-ple different effects, so that the effects of evolutionary change are not restricted to any bounded and non-porous psychological faculty, but are instead complex and multi-levelled (so there is unlikely to be "a gene" that explains language in humans). Furthermore, such genetic and behavioural changes need to be understood within ever-changing gene–environment contexts; a particular change may be bad for the par-ticular individual at a particular time, but nevertheless be selected for because it is good for some individuals at some times (e.g. the gene that increases various impulsive traits including susceptibility to alcoholism (Gerard & Higley, 2002) and perhaps infidelity).

The debate within evolutionary psychology about "spandrels" – by-products of evolution that cannot properly be considered to be functions – provides a test case for a more integrative approach to evolu-tionary explanation. Gould famously pointed out that although humans developed a large brain in response to adaptive pressures, the many by-products of large brains (e.g. music, religion, writing) should not properly be explained in terms of functions (Gould, 1991).[16] Thus evo-lutionary psychology cannot rely solely on explanations of adaptation, but also requires an understanding of so-called exaptation. Buss and col-leagues (1998) have countered that there are criteria that can be applied to the assessment of explanations, whether or not these are explicitly evolutionary, and whether they involve an adaptation or an exaptation. From the integrative perspective taken here, the point is not so much whether there has been adaptation or exaptation, but rather whether cognitive-affective functions can be explained in terms of the relevant underlying structures and mechanisms. Complex cognitive-affective processes such as language and infidelity may need to be understood less in terms of rule-based evolved modules, and more as emergent

---

[16] Gould criticizes a reductionistic view of evolutionary theory, which he terms "Darwinian fundamentalism". Certainly, a range of non-reductionist approaches have been put forward in evolutionary theory, for example, emphasizing gene–culture coevolution (Cavalli-Sforza & Feldman, 1981) and niche construction (Olding-Smee *et al.*, 2003).

properties of humans with brain-minds living in societies (Panksepp & Panksepp, 2000).

Put differently, at the more general level of a philosophical consideration of functions and evolutionary theory (Boorse, 1976b; Davies, 2003; Dennett, 1995; Fulford, 1999, 2001; Hempel, 1965; Mayr, 1988; Megone, 2000; Millikan, 1984; Ruse, 1971; Sadler & Agich, 1995; Thornton, 2000; Wright, 1976), it can be argued that the very concepts of "function" and "dysfunction", and particularly human cognitive-affective function and dysfunction, cannot be specified in a classical way in terms of necessary and sufficient conditions, but rather require more powerful explanations that address particular aspects of their embodiment and context. In line with the earlier example of sickle cell anaemia, let us say that there are brain-mind mechanisms which mean, during exposure to a particularly well-resourced environment, that mood is more narrowly regulated, but that during exposure to a more adverse environment mood becomes more responsive to stressors. Mood instability may be a brain-mind "dysfunction" only insofar as the organism later lives in a well-resourced environment, but it may be an adaptation in stressful environments where more risky strategies are beneficial. Furthermore, when it comes to considering people, brain-minds have evolved to interact with complex social environments, so that explanations of how brain-mind phenomena and processes are adaptive or not, or working well or not, are particularly likely to have to move beyond a consideration solely of body-brain mechanisms, to consider also human practices and values. The term "dysfunction" often represents an oversimplification; in typical cases it usefully overlaps with our common metaphors of disorder and serves as a convenient explanation, but in many other cases a detailed understanding of the relevant (psychobiological) structures and mechanisms, and of the interactive context in which they operate, is important for a full understanding (of psychopathology).[17]

---

[17] Parallel considerations may apply to how we think of evolution in general. Some evolutionary theorists have blurred the notion between fitness and goodness, seeing evolution as progressive. Darwin himself rarely used the term "evolution", instead speaking of "descent with variation", and emphasizing that variations are random and not necessarily progressive (Ruse, 2003).

This is not to say, however, that evolutionary theory is unhelpful in contributing to questions about human nature in general (Millikan, 1984; Papineau, 1993) and disorder in particular (Cosmides & Tooby, 1999; Mealey, 1997; Nesse, 2001). As noted above, by emphasizing context, an evolutionary perspective has highlighted "mismatch" between current behaviour and behaviour that evolved within the environment of evolutionary adaptedness (EEA) (Bowlby, 1980). In our own context of the twenty-first century, we need to decide as best we can how to intervene when such a mismatch occurs. Ageing may have been functional in the EEA, but in the twenty-first century it may well be entirely reasonable to lower our threshold for making ageing-related diagnoses and treating accordingly. At the other end of the age spectrum, childhood attention deficit/hyperactivity disorder may not involve a design deficit (as evolution makes space for genes that code for impulsivity), but in the context of modern educational requirements and available treatments, such a diagnosis may be considered valid. For Wakefield, alcoholism may not be a disorder given the absence of an underlying design deficit, but for clinicians working in the context of contemporary societies, it provides an extremely useful and entirely valid metaphor – alcoholism is not merely a sin or a crime, and it has much in common with more prototypic medical disorders.

In summary, in order to understand fully the nature of a disorder, we need not only knowledge about the adaptation of particular psychobiological mechanisms over evolutionary time, but also a range of other information, including information about the relevant underlying structures and mechanisms, and the relevant context in which they operate. Evolutionary theories may propose, for example, that social anxiety is maladaptive (insofar as it is associated with decreased fertility) or adaptive (in that it promotes social awareness), but whether or not we explain social anxiety in terms of a disorder (seeing social anxiety, metaphorically, as reflecting an imbalance, a breakdown, etc.), in fact depends on a range of other considerations (such as the distress and impairment associated with symptoms within a particular cultural and historical period). Evolutionary theory is nevertheless useful insofar as it sheds light on how a range of different phenomena can be maladaptive (Cosmides & Tooby, 1999; Mealey, 1997; Nesse, 2001), and provides insights into the mechanisms that underpin such phenomena. Furthermore, as evolutionary theory progresses, and as relevant empirical data accumulate, this may contribute in part to changing our ideas about the mapping of a particular condition within the prototypic categories of disorder, and about using the prototypic explanation of dysfunction.

6

Moral questions about psychotropics

In this chapter we address a series of questions about ethical choices. The classical versus critical contrast drawn throughout this volume can perhaps also be applied to ethics. A classical approach would take the view that decisions about ethics in general and bioethics[1] in particular can be made on the basis of moral laws. Thinkers from Plato to Kant have described the rationality of such universal and fixed rules, with more recent philosophers such as Rawls (1971) viewing moral theory as a kind of grammar. In contrast, a critical position emphasizes that such a view is unrealizable given that decisions about ethics and bioethics reflect the concerns and values of the particular historical and geographical contexts in which they are made. Hegel, for example, argued that a systems of laws loses its meaning when attempts are made to abstract it from its grounding in the ethical life of a particular historical community.

Here a realist, naturalist, and embodied position is taken, arguing that insofar as decisions about ethics and bioethics are informed by universal biologically based considerations, there exists the potential for minimal standards of agreement about ethics and about values, and it is possible to debate reasonably (cognitively–affectively) in order to ensure that good bioethics decisions are reached.[2] Thus, for example, there is

---

[1] The term "bioethics" was coined by Potter (1971). For a history of how bioethics was given impetus by new technologies such as organ transplantation and mechanical ventilation see, for example, Rothman (1991) and Jonsen (2000).

[2] The term "naturalist" requires some unpacking here. Moore famously argued that the attempt to define goodness in descriptive terms commits the "naturalistic fallacy" (Moore,

near-universal agreement that when physicians relieve pain this is a good thing, and it is also possible to argue reasonably for the importance of not relieving pain or suffering in particular contexts (Barris, 1990; De Botton, 2001; Johnson, 1993) or, conversely, that there has been under-medication of pain in certain circumstances. The aim of the chapter is not to argue for this last approach in its own terms, but rather to use this framework to put forward a position on three important ethical questions in psychopharmacology, namely: (1) is treatment of psychiatric disorder a good thing?, (2) is pharmacotherapy a good kind of intervention?, and (3) is pharmacotherapy for enhanced performance a good thing?

Is treatment of psychiatric disorder a good thing?

The idea that there might be a single overarching value or conception of human flourishing seems highly improbable in light of the diversity of our needs, desires, and practices. (Johnson, 1993)

To those human beings who are of any concern to me I wish suffering, desolation, sickness, ill-treatment, indignities. (Nietzche, 1968)

Injari Imsingh visited his doctor after feeling stressed out at work. He noted that there had been conflict there about schedule planning, and that he felt humiliated by his supervisor and co-workers. He wanted a medication to help him sleep better. This would be for a short time, as the Human Resources Department had agreed to mediate the situation soon. On further questioning, he admitted to severe symptoms of depression.

1903). In opposition, some continue to propose a concept of "natural" good, that depends, for example, on facts about one's species (Foot, 2003; Hursthouse, 1999). In defending a naturalist virtue based ethics, MacIntyre traces such a position back to Aristotle, who, as a biologist, attempted to give an account of the good that was both local and particular, and yet also cosmic and universal (MacIntyre, 1981). A range of writers fall on the spectrum between a broader moral naturalism (which holds that a naturalist approach to philosophical inquiry in general is adequate for moral philosophy) and a narrower moral naturalism (which holds that there are natural moral facts and properties). The approach developed in this volume is to highlight the complexity of facts about the human species and the way these interact with human values, consistent with a non-reductionistic naturalism.

However, when the option of referral to a psychiatrist for treatment was discussed, he stated that if he took such a step, then this would mean that his colleagues had truly defeated him. He indicated that he really wanted the mediation process to work in his favour; he felt that this was the key step towards feeling less humiliated. He also believed that his corporation was an essentially inhumane one, in which individuals could not truly flourish. There was little chance that he would ever advance beyond his current, rather inferior, position in the company.

A classical perspective on the concept and explanation of disorder may regard depression as a disorder because it is characterized by dysfunction. Symptoms of this disorder include negatively biased cognitive distortions about the self, about the world, and about the future, and these are then an appropriate focus of treatment. Cognitive therapy, for example, aims to change cognitive distortions, so that a person is able to function more realistically and more happily in the world. Cognitive therapy relies on an alliance between clinician and patient, and an agreement to examine closely the data of the world. When this is done in therapy, it turns out that negative thinking about the self, the world, and the future can be shown to be unrealistic. This exploration gradually persuades the patient to think more clearly, and so to develop a more positive outlook on the self, the world, and the future.

A critical perspective on the concept and explanation of symptoms may, however, emphasize normal variations in mood, the possibility that some events are so horrific that depression seems a reasonable response (Elliott, 2007),[3] and the phenomenon of "depressive realism" (people with depressive symptoms can in fact be more realistic about a number of things, such as judging contingencies between their responses and subsequent outcomes (Haaga & Beck, 1995)). Thus it has been argued that the depressive "has a keener eye for the truth" (Freud, 1917), and that "depressives' thoughts are painfully truthful, whereas

---

[3] Elliott gives the example of Sisyphus on Prozac; he argues that even if Sisyphus appreciated the prescription, this would not mean he had a mental health problem, as given that he will be pushing a boulder up the mountain for eternity, alienation is an appropriate response. Conversely, he argues that some lives are better than other lives, regardless of the psychological well-being of the people who are living them (Elliott, 2007).

non-depressives' thoughts are unrealistically positive" (Layne, 1983). Aristotle, Heidegger and others have famously argued that depression and anxiety can lead to philosophical insights (Graham, 1990; Radden, 2000; Simon, 1978; Svenaeus, 2007).[4] The fact of depressive realism demonstrates that cognitive therapy is not at all "scientific" in its methods or "objective" in its goals. Rather, therapy is a way of persuading patients to conform to social practices. Societies are characterized by particular ideologies, and these may include overly optimistic views of the world and its future. Psychotherapy, like other medical interventions, promotes the ideology of a particular time and place, reduces social deviance, and may well diminish creativity.

Analogous positions on a range of psychiatric disorders and symptoms can be found in the bioethics literature. A classical position, for example, argues that where medical conditions (e.g. social anxiety disorder) involve dysfunction, then they are disorders deserving of treatment (Sabin & Daniels, 1994). This position may rely on necessary and sufficient definitions of important terms (such as the term "person" in debate on abortion) (Goldman, 1993a; Johnson, 1993; Stich, 1993), or may attempt to strictly parse the descriptive and evaluative components of a particular construct (such as "disorder"; Wakefield, 1992a; Williams, 1985).[5] Further, in this position, applied ethics in general, and bioethics in particular, is able to justify its prescriptions in terms of the rational application of moral theories to medical situations (Hedgecoe, 2004; Rawls, 1971).

On the basis of a determination about whether a relevant condition involves, say, a dysfunction (a matter of fact), and a determination about whether, say, maximum benefit for the community is being achieved (a matter of value), for example, a principled decision can be made

---

[4] Indeed, Camus has claimed that suicide is the only serious philosophical question. In a more light-hearted vein, Bentall has built on such claims and proposed that happiness is a psychiatric disorder (Bentall, 1992).

[5] Questions about the is–ought distinction date at least back to Hume (1739). As noted in a previous footnote, Moore (1903) made an influential case against ethical naturalism. Ayer later wrote, "We hold that one really never does dispute about questions of value" (1936), while Hare (1952) distinguished between descriptive and evaluative expressions. Ironically, this denial of the role of reason in moral debate means that there is a thread of relativism running from Moore's intuitionism to contemporary emotivism (MacIntyre, 1981).

as to whether or not to treat. In this classic view, modern bioethics is able to resolve questions raised by the practice of medicine, including problems raised by new technologies, by means of moral rules, which apply universally (Macklin, 1999), and sustain the important distinction between facts and values. An influential form of principle-based ethics or principlism (Beauchamp & Childress, 2001) has attempted to reconcile deontological rules (such as those proposed by Kant (1785)) and duty-based ethics with utilitarian rules (such as those proposed by Mill (1863)) and a consequentialist ethics, by emphasizing "mid-level" principles that are subject to change depending on the relevant context.

In contrast, a critical position may argue that emotional distress (e.g. anxiety in social situations, suffering after trauma) is often a normal and even valuable phenomenon (Tedeschi *et al.*, 1998), that our constructs (or "idioms") of distress are culture-bound (Young, 1995), and that such distress need not necessarily be medicalized (Kleinman, 1988). Increased prescriptions of psychotropics for emotions in women may reflect an unwarranted pathologizing of femininity (Hamilton *et al.*, 1995; Metzl, 2003). Application of the Western construct of social anxiety disorder in the East, where people instead experience *taijin kyofusho* (worry about offending others) or *lek* (fear of disrupting one's cultural role in a social performance), and insistence on Western treatment, may be inappropriate. This position emphasizes that decisions about ethics and bioethics reflect the concerns and values of the particular historical and geographical contexts in which they are made. Part of the meaning of particular words (such as "person"), is a certain moral attitude (Elliott, 1999; Johnston, 1989). Certainly, a close examination of the words and metaphors used in moral reasoning (Johnson, 1993; Putnam, 2002) and of the nature of bioethics (Alderson, 1990; Bosk, 1992; DeVries & Subedi, 1998; Elliott, 1999; Evans, 2002; Fox & Swazey, 1992; Hoffmaster, 2000; Komesaroff, 1995; Lock & Kaufert, 1998; Shildrick & Mykitiuk, 2005; Stevens, 2000) seem to refute the notion of a fact–value distinction.

From a critical perspective, therefore, there is a need for bioethical principlism to be replaced by approaches such as narrative, pragmatic, and critical ethics (Chambers, 1999; Eldridge, 1989; Frank, 1979;

Gardner, 1978; Hedgecoe, 2004; MacIntyre, 1981; McGee, 1997; Nelson, 1997; Nussbaum, 1990; Toulmin, 2001; Zaner, 1993). One well-known approach, known as care ethics, argues that rules such as the deontological emphasis on autonomy, or the utilitarian focus on impartiality, ignore the interpersonal dimension of moral life (Baier, 1985). Given that no principle can claim primacy in a society characterized by diverse moral views, it instead draws on Aristotelean theory in calling for the cultivation of virtuous traits such as sympathy and compassion to promote ethical clinical behaviour, and emphasizes Hume's argument that ethical behaviour derives from these kinds of sentiment (Bloch & Green, 2006).

This volume cannot adequately cover the large philosophical literature that has debated these issues. Consistent with the approach taken throughout, a position that is able to avoid classic concepts of categories, but at the same time not slide into the relativism of some critical thinkers, would be attractive (Johnson, 1993; Lovibond, 1983; Williams, 1985). Similarly, a position that allowed a space for cognitive–affective science within ethical thinking, would be appealing (Goldman, 1993a; Williams, 1985). Various writers on the values and ethics of psychiatry have attempted to formulate a position that balances objectivism and subjectivism (Bloch & Green, 2006; Thornton, 2000). However, again in keeping with the approach throughout the volume, rather than attempt to defend such a position on its own terms, we will first turn to the data, to see whether these can help sustain such a position. In the relatively simple case of whether to treat psychiatric disorder, the data do seem informative. In later parts of the chapter, more subtle questions are addressed, and there are arguably fewer data available.

What do the data from cognitive–affective science reveal about whether or not to treat depression in particular, and psychiatric disorder in general? Our cognitive–affective maps allow us to reason precisely and accurately about the physical world, and the instruments of science (e.g. microscopy, telescopy) have extended our knowledge of its structures and mechanisms (Giere, 1988). Indeed, our sensorimotor-affective systems arguably evolved in order to help us function in the physical and social world (Duchaine *et al.*, 2001). On the other hand, our cognitive–affective maps are also designed to make sure that we function effectively in the social world, and this may require that we are unrealistically optimistic in some respects (Goleman, 1996). For example, we need to devote extraordinary resources to our offspring, and believe that this will reap happiness for us, whereas bringing up children is in fact a risky and not necessarily productive endeavour.

From this kind of data and theory about human brain-minds, there is no reason why we should have evolved to be happy with our lot; instead, people who are always striving for more resources may have an advantage when circumstances change and they are able to use their surplus stock. A certain amount of depressive realism may be particularly adaptive under some circumstances – for example, when our strategies require rethinking (Nesse, 2000). Nevertheless, there is also a good deal of evidence to support the idea that once symptoms of depression have achieved a particular level of severity, then compared with healthy volunteers, patients demonstrate marked changes in their underlying neurocircuitry, neurochemistry, and cognitive–affective processes (Stein, 2003; Stein *et al.*, 2006). Thus, we can develop sophisticated causal classifications of depression, based on a nuanced understanding of the interaction of biology and culture (Hansen & Maynes, 2005).

Furthermore, there is a good deal of clinical data demonstrating that when patients meet criteria for major depression and have clinical distress, they then suffer from significant impairment (e.g. in social, occupational, and family functioning). In addition, there is a good deal of clinical data showing that various psychiatric interventions, including both pharmacotherapy and psychotherapy, can reduce depressive symptoms, that such improvement is accompanied by normalization of neurocircuitry and neurochemistry, by changes in cognitive–affective processes, and by reduced distress and impairment. Thus appropriate psychiatric treatment can help patients lead "good lives" (Reznek, 1991). Finally, when depression has a particular level of severity and impairment then such an outcome can be achieved cost-effectively (Chisholm *et al.*, 2004).

Thus it seems that there is the possibility that medical decision-making, such as a decision to treat a case of depression, even though value-laden, can usefully be informed by scientific data (Haimes, 2002; Hedgecoe, 2004). It is notable that patients who have to make such decisions appear to rely less on classical constructs (such as disorder), and more on real-world impacts (Rapp, 2000). People choose a particular ethical rule to apply based not on universal principles, but rather on the particularity of their specific interests and values (Alderson, 1990). Rather than attempt to find a neutral answer to all similar cases, it is more reasonable to refine our bioethical reasoning by examining empirically how medical decision-making works, and by reflexively refining the constructs and methods which underpin such decision-making (Hedgecoe, 2004). More broadly, although we can perhaps expect diversity rather than convergence in moral reasoning (Hampshire, 1983), and certainly ongoing debate about the nature of human nature in general, good reasons can be found for a particular individual to make specific choices in life (Johnson, 1993; Williams, 1985).

Are there any data to support the argument that although medical decision-making appears to involve both facts and values (Canguilhem, 1966; de Beaufort *et al.*, 2000; Fulford, 1989; Fulford *et al.*, 2005; Hare, 1983; Pellegrino & Thomasma, 1981; Sadler, 1997, 2002; Schaffner, 1999; Wakefield, 1992b), it can nevertheless be reasonable? Certainly, there is growing interest in empirical work on the cognitive–affective science of decision-making in general and of medical decision-making in particular. It is notable that such work demonstrates a range of important biases in human cognitive–affective processes, including biases in judging values (Ainslie, 2001; Baumeister *et al.*, 2001; Kahneman & Tversky, 2000; Piatelli-Palmarini, 1994). At the same time, humans are experts at weighing up human practices and interests; accurate evaluation of such phenomena is key to our success in social interactions. And it can be argued that as our understanding of the mechanisms underlying medical decision-making improves, so our ability to reach better decisions will also potentially be enhanced (although this proposal remains to be fully demonstrated).

With this research on human brain-minds and their decision-making in mind, we can return to the case outlined above. Although Injari's depression may well be a consequence of circumstances at work, it can reasonably be considered a medical disorder that deserves treatment. We may not be able to rely on an evolutionary theory of dysfunction (see above), or on algorithmic ethical principles, to define when depressive symptoms should be characterized as a disorder and treatment initiated. Rather, this is a clinical decision which includes a range of considerations, including our explanation of the relevant proximal (psychobiological) and distal (evolutionary) mechanisms, our understanding of the extent of suffering and impairment of the individual patient, and our consideration of the efficacy and cost-effectiveness of possible intervention.

It may be countered that the argument here is somewhat disingenuous in that depression is a more typical disorder (which is disvalued), so that any conclusions about the benefit of data on treatments which show a reduction in symptoms (which is valued) is tautological. As suggested earlier, judgements about the typicality of disorders may reflect universal biologically based considerations; an acute infection, for example, may occur in a previously healthy person and severely disrupt body function, and in this instance there is little disagreement from place to place, and time to time, that this would represent a medical condition deserving of treatment. Similarly, although the classical and critical approaches might differ in their views of depression, both a lay and a scientific view can readily converge on the conclusion that this is a medical disorder that deserves treatment. We have previously referred to other psychiatric conditions, however, which have more atypical features, and where the term "disorder" is therefore more contentious, namely social anxiety disorder and impulsivity. Are these deserving of psychiatric treatment?

Although we can posit that social anxiety disorder is indicative of pathological activation of a normal social anxiety alarm, there may well be a continuum between variation in normal personality traits and this condition, and in any particular individual any assertion about the presence of a disease process can only be inferred. On the other hand, there is a growing range of data indicating that the experience of severe social anxiety in both the West (social anxiety disorder) and East (*taijin kyofusho*) is mediated by overlapping psychobiological mechanisms, is accompanied by significant distress and impairment, and responds effectively and cost-effectively to the same class of medication (Stein & Matsunaga, 2001). Thus, in the realist compromise outlined in this volume, social anxiety disorder and *taijin kyofusho* are validly considered as related disorders, and it is reasonable to treat them with psychiatric interventions, albeit bearing in mind differences in the way social anxiety is expressed and experienced in different contexts (Stein & Matsunaga, 2001).

This is not to say that we should treat all socially anxious individuals, but it is to argue that promotion of awareness of this diagnosis and of its treatment is reasonable. Murray Stein, an expert on social anxiety disorder, asks the question, "Are we needlessly 'medicalising' a normal variant of temperament, performing cosmetic psychopharmacology to remove blemishes of the personality?" (Stein, 1996b). He and other psychiatrists working in the area answer with an emphatic no, emphasizing factors such as the growing understanding of the psychobiology of social anxiety disorder, the associated distress and impairment, and the availability of effective and cost-effective treatments (Campbell-Sills & Stein, 2005). Wakefield and colleagues argue that most cases of social anxiety disorder should not be understood as disorder, but nevertheless agree that social anxiety can be accompanied by enormous suffering, and that those who have such anxiety deserve clinical attention as a matter of compassion and justice (Wakefield *et al.*, 2005).

What about impulsivity? Does impulsive-aggression, for example, merely represent a spectrum of deviant behaviour, for which the person must take responsibility, and which falls under the jurisdiction of the law and the church, or should it be considered a medical disorder (intermittent explosive disorder, in DSM-IV-TR) that deserves treatment (Duff, 1986; Elliott, 1996; Flew, 1973; Glover, 1970; Hart, 1968; Lucas, 1993; Tam, 1996)?[6] As we discover more about the subtle psychobiological alterations underlying impulsive behaviours (including those characteristic of substance use disorders and so-called behavioural addictions), learn more about the disability associated with this impulsivity and its psychobiological correlates, and develop more effective and cost-effective medical interventions that normalize this psychobiology,

---

[6] Here one is reminded of Samuel Butler's "Erewhon", where criminals are treated as ill, and vice versa. This book is also one of the first to write about the possibility that machines develop consciousness.

decrease impulsive behaviours, and improve impairment, then it may well become increasingly sensible to medicalize some of these behaviours.

At the same time, optimal interventions for decreasing impulsivity do seem to include an emphasis on accepting personal responsibility and on the importance of social limits and boundaries (whether instantiated in the therapeutic milieu, or in the structures of the justice system). In the case of antisocial personality disorder, even though psychobiological disturbances may well be present, medical interventions are also singularly unimpressive in efficacy. Thus, an individualized approach again seems necessary; for a particular person at a particular time, psychiatric treatment may be a justifiable intervention to decrease impulsive-aggression (Stein, 1994, 1996a), but in other cases there is also a reasonable role for interventions such as legal sanction (Dennett, 2003; Garland, 2004; Greene & Cohen, 2004; Masters & McGuire, 1994; McCall Smith, 2004; Morse, 2006; Reznek, 1997).[7] Psychiatric research aims to provide better prognosticators of what intervention will work optimally for whom.

Is pharmacotherapy a good kind of intervention?

Now, it is to retreat before stress, and to reject one's responsibilities to ask a drug to create indifference and oblivion in the face of one's duties; this is a fatal renunciation which can only end in compromises and failure. (Pope Pius XII)

People who fall back on rules and moral laws are people who are either afraid of the indeterminancy and contingency of life, or morally obtuse, or both. (Johnson, 1993)

Injari's mediation went poorly for him. He was told that he must accept the work scheduling as developed by his supervisor and agreed to by his

---

[7] The philosophical literature on concepts such as free will, determinism, autonomy, and responsibility is too large to review here. In general, the approach here is consistent with a compatabilist view, which emphasizes degrees of freedom. Similarly, an approach that balances different accounts and consequences may be relevant for thinking about weakness of will, or akrasia (Davidson, 1984; Williams, 1985).

colleagues. Given the increased severity of his depressive symptoms, he agreed to take an antidepressant. Within a few weeks he felt significantly better. A few months later he reported that not only had his earlier depression resolved, but that he was thinking about his work in an entirely different way. He felt that his corporation was really rather a good one, and that Human Resources had gone out of their way to establish programmes to help individuals to grow and develop. He felt optimistic about his future in the company, and believed that with some luck he could progress up the corporate ladder.

If judgements about the disvalue of disorders, and about the benefit of treatment, reflect universal biologically based considerations, then as noted in the previous section, there is likely to be a good deal of consensus about the value of such intervention, particularly when the disorders, and their treatments, are more typical in nature. In the last section, we briefly considered some atypical disorders. In this section and the next, we focus on different kinds of treatments. Our first question is whether pharmacotherapy can be justified, given the availability of other kinds of interventions, which may be viewed as more conventional ways of acting to alter disturbed behaviour. Thus, if a psychiatric disorder can be treated with two equally effective interventions, one a pharmacotherapy and another a psychotherapy, which one should be used as a first-line strategy? And what if a psychiatric disorder can be overcome with entirely non-medical interventions, such as more exercise, or prayer; should these not be the approach of choice?

In the classical position different therapeutic options can be evaluated with the data at hand; this might include direct comparisons of two different modalities of intervention on symptom reduction, or examination of other kinds of data such as the economic costs of treatment. Evidence-based medicine provides a range of scientific methodologies for undertaking such comparisons, and it turns out there is good data for efficacy and cost-efficacy for pharmacotherapy, for cognitive-behavioural psychotherapy, and even for exercise for a number of psychiatric disorders. In these cases, then, the choice of treatment modality becomes a matter of physician capability and of patient preference.

There is no reason not to be optimistic about future progress in biotechnology (Buchanan *et al.*, 2000; Resnik *et al.*, 1999; Stock, 2002).

The critical position highlights, however, that different kinds of intervention have different kinds of meaning, and therefore different consequences, for different people. Some might view medication as merely a quick and superficial fix for behavioural problems, and would prefer the personal growth offered by an insight-oriented psychotherapy. After all, some have defined psychoanalysis as "the search for truth about oneself". Others might, however, regard cognitive-behavioural psychotherapy, which aims at decreasing symptoms rather than at self-discovery as the most appropriate kind of psychotherapy. Indeed, some argue that a contemporary "culture of therapy" has led to an abdication of moral responsibility in favour of self-obsession and self-absorption (Rosen, 1977; Sommers & Satel, 2004). For others still, non-medical interventions are invariably a preferred choice. To focus only on the "thin" technological endpoints of symptom recovery misses the "thick" process whereby the method used to achieve change has a range of other consequences, and the particular values of psychotherapy (Cole-Turner, 1998; Goldberg, 2007; Holmes & Lindley, 1989; Rieff, 1979).

The meaning of any particular intervention in turn reflects the relevant historical and cultural context. In the twenty-first century, where science and technology have such powerful positive connotations, many of us have a growing trust in and reliance on medical technologies and medication, including psychotropics. Modern medication has major advantages, not only directly because of its efficacy and cost-effectiveness, but also indirectly by emphasizing the biological component of psychiatric disorders, encouraging suffers to talk openly about their illness, and facilitating a humane medical approach to those with brain-mind disorders (whose deviant behaviour may otherwise be classified as illegal or as evil; Reznek, 1991; Stein & Gureje, 2004).

Increasingly, consumer advocacy groups with an interest in psychiatric disorders such as depression argue that such conditions are "brain disorders", and lobby for increased availability of psychiatric medications. They argue for the importance of increased mental health literacy amongst the population at large (Jorm, 2000), hoping that greater knowledge of the neurobiology of psychiatric disorders will help lower the multiple individual and social barriers to seeking help (Seedat *et al.*, 2002), and lead to improved diagnosis and earlier treatment. This view has the potential advantage of emphasizing that psychiatric disorders are medical disorders, and of therefore increasing resources for these conditions as well as decreasing the enormous stigmatization that is associated with suffering from a psychiatric disorder and with receiving treatment with psychiatric agents.

On the other hand, there have also been warnings from some philosophers about the dangers of technology (Heidegger, 1999), and our era is characterized by a strong view that medical technologies have a dehumanizing element and do not provide us with a sufficient sense of meaning (Bullard, 2002; Dworkin, 2006; Fukuyama, 2002; Greenhalgh & Hurwitz, 1998; Kriel, 2000; Schwartz & Wiggins, 1986). This view is associated with a wariness about relying on medication in general, and psychotropics in particular. The pharmacological management of our mental lives threatens to confer on us "a fraudulent happiness" and to be character-deforming (President's Council on Bioethics, 2003). Medicalization does not necessarily lead to a lack of stigma (e.g. people with HIV are often found blameworthy). Disease mongering has important disadvantages, including iatrogenic harm (from adverse events associated with medication) and wasting of resources (Moynihan & Henry, 2006), while over-medicalization leads to indirect problems such as the neglect of socio-political factors in explaining and combating ill health and prioritizing the wrong kinds of health care research (Callahan, 2003).

The notion that psychiatric medication should be used as sparingly as possible has been termed "pharmacological Calvinism" (Klerman, 1972). To extend the quotation above of one (Catholic) authority,

Life every day brings burdens and problems which must be confronted with lucidity, and resolved with Christian faith and wisdom. Now, it is to retreat before stress, and to reject one's responsibilities to ask a drug to create indifference and oblivion in the face of one's duties; this is a fatal renunciation which can only end in compromises and failure. An anxiety must take care of itself, mobilizing its strength to draw up plans and bring realistic behaviour to a successful conclusion, whereby the Christian derives something from faith, hope, and charity. (Thullier, 1999)

Such a view has the potential advantage of helping to prevent inappropriate overoptimism about psychotropics (for example, the introduction of barbiturates was accompanied by publicity about "happy pills" and "aspirin for the soul" despite their significant adverse events (Smith, 1991)).

Following the approach taken throughout this volume, an integrative perspective would be wary of any attempt to find a universal rule that judged some therapeutic modality better than others, or that rejected the possibility of any reasonable decision about the relative value of different modalities. A key point is that for any particular individual, a great deal of conceptual and empirical work may be required to determine what the best intervention is, at any particular point in time. Further, in some cases, the best psychiatric intervention may in fact be no psychiatric treatment (Frances & Clarkin, 1981). During the course of psychiatric evaluation and intervention, the clinician ought to make every effort to understand the patient, from the perspective of both (psychobiological) mechanisms and (personal) meanings, to consider carefully whether pharmacotherapy and/or psychotherapy is the best choice, and then to evaluate empirically the effects of such intervention. Whether or not medication is used in an authentic way depends not simply on the medication itself, but on the context in which it is administered.

Do the data from cognitive–affective science support such a stance? Cognitive–affective science is always interested in the relevant underlying mechanisms. Looking at the neuronal circuitry which mediates psychopathology, as described in the previous chapter, it seems clear that both particular medications and specific psychotherapies can alter neurocircuitry and effectively reduce psychiatric symptoms (Baxter *et al.*, 1992; Furmark *et al.*, 2002; Paquetta *et al.*, 2003; Roffman *et al.*, 2005; Straube *et al.*, 2006). It turns out that exercise and prayer also have powerful brain-mind effects. However, brain imaging data also show different predictors of response to different modalities (for example, in obsessive–compulsive disorder, decreased frontal activity is a positive predictor of response to medication, but a negative predictor of response to psychotherapy; Brody *et al.*, 1998). In addition, different treatment modalities are experienced in entirely different ways by different

people, and there is a growing understanding of the relevant mechanisms (as alluded to in the earlier discussion of the placebo response).

Indeed, in psychiatric practice, a range of different modalities are
used, not so much because such a strategy is evidence-based (i.e.
based on data from studies comparing different modalities), but rather
because each modality has distinct advantages and disadvantages for
particular individuals. As noted earlier, it is also often a useful clinical strategy to not only investigate symptoms and their underpinnings
(the disease), but to also explore the person's understanding of their experience (the illness) (Kleinman, 1988; Stein, 1993). A decision can then
be negotiated between clinician and patient that takes into account not
only the scientific data on treatment, but also the meaning of particular interventions. Thus, for a particular person, in a particular context,
pharmacotherapy (or psychotherapy, or a decision not to employ psychiatric treatment) may be an optimal psychiatric intervention.[8]

Returning to the case of Injari, while psychotherapy might well have
been useful in addressing his conflicts at work, a model focused on
medication turned out to be acceptable and effective. More generally,
in clinical practice, it can be argued that it is paramount to understand
each individual that presents for treatment, and to try to choose the best
intervention for a particular person at a particular time. This position is
one that goes beyond the views that medical decision-making involves
merely a consideration of the observable data of the universe in general
and of the world of clinical trials in particular (the classical position), or
that medical decision-making is merely reflective of a particular time
and place and therefore entirely subjective or relativistic (the critical
position). In particular circumstances, either pharmacotherapy or psychotherapy can be an "authentic" choice (Elliott, 2003) that is in the
best interests of the patient.

What about cases where psychological mechanisms appear
paramount? Certainly, in cases where exposure to psychological trauma
has led to PTSD, clinical tradition has emphasized the value of

---

[8] Notably, there is a growing empirical literature investigating the predictors of different
explanatory models of disorder and attitudes towards pharmacotherapy (Horne *et al.*, 2004),
the effects of such models and attitudes on outcomes (Garfield *et al.*, 2003; Lam *et al.*, 2005),
and the impact of new psychotropics on such models and attitudes (Metzl & Angel, 2004).

psychotherapeutic intervention. There is a literature which emphasizes that suffering after severe psychological trauma is better understood as a meaningful response to an abnormal event than as a disorder, and which notes that a meaningful psychosocial response can lead to healing and even to posttraumatic psychological growth (Tedeschi & McFarlare, 1998). Nevertheless, a more recent literature emphasizes that PTSD, like other psychiatric disorders, involves a range of vulnerability factors, and is characterized by psychobiological disruption (Rauch *et al.*, 1998; Yehuda & McFarlane, 1995). There is a growing literature which indicates that both pharmacotherapy and psychotherapy can be useful in people with PTSD.

Counter-intuitively, in the immediate aftermath of exposure to psychological trauma, debriefing is ineffective (Rose *et al.*, 2002), while pharmacotherapy may help prevent PTSD (Pitman *et al.*, 2002). Although additional empirical work is clearly needed in this area (Glannon, 2006b; Henry *et al.*, 2007), the ethics of erasing painful memories have already been questioned (President's Council on Bioethics, 2003). Certainly, there are good reasons for emphasizing that after exposure to trauma, we should emphasize that psychiatric symptoms are typically transient, and encourage resilience and bravery (Stein *et al.*, 2007). At the same time, the general argument put forward here, emphasizing the potential value of pharmacotherapy in certain individuals (for example, those who are at particularly high-risk for developing PTSD), may well apply.

Importantly, however, in the practice of good psychiatry, it is false to contrast a scientific pharmacotherapy with non-scientific psychotherapy. Good pharmacotherapy requires a sensitive understanding of the other person (and therefore may evoke a placebo response). Good psychotherapy is based on a scientific knowledge of the empirical database of psychotherapy studies, and of explanations about how particular cognitive–affective schemas act to disrupt personal relationships, including the doctor–patient relationship (which may therefore evoke a nocebo response). There is no universal rule about pharmacotherapy that can decide between the black and white choices of utopian optimism and dystopian Calvinism, between epicurean pill-popping and stoic denial; rather, each case must be judged on its merits, which may involve many subtle shades of grey.

As Peter Kramer (1997) writes, "Pharmacotherapy, when looked at closely, will appear to be as arbitrary – as much an art, not least in the derogatory sense of being impressionistic where ideally it should be objective – as psychotherapy. Like any other serious assessment of human emotional life, pharmacotherapy rests on fallible attempts at intimate understanding of another person".[9] Phrased in a more positive way, both pharmacotherapy and psychotherapy (Engelhardt, 1973) involve a doctor–patient relationship in which there is an attempt to understand the patient, not solely as an object of technical manipulation, but also as a person, and to determine what is best for him or her. It is no accident, then, that considerations not only about the role of reason, but also about the importance of empathy, lie at the heart of so much thinking on both psychiatric care (Stein, 2005), and moral philosophy (Blum, 1980; Flanagan, 1991; Goldman, 1993a; Hare, 1963; Hume, 1739; Rawls, 1971; Schopenhauer, 1965; Smith, 2002).

Is pharmacotherapy for enhanced performance a good thing?

And if ever, by some unlucky chance, anything unpleasant should happen, why, there's always soma to give a holiday from the facts. And there's always soma to calm your anger, to reconcile you to your enemies, to make you patient and long-suffering. In the past you could only accomplish these things by making a great effort and after years of moral training. Now, you swallow two or three half-gramme tablets, and there you are. Anybody can be virtuous now. (Huxley, 1932)

Most people in Pala take the moksha medicine only a few times a year, and its effects are compared to those of meditation – a practice which has an important place in everyday Palanese life... Both meditation and moksha-medicine improve social intelligence, self-knowledge, and self-understanding... moksha-medicine helps one by 'getting to know oneself to the point where one won't be compelled by one's unconscious to do all the ugly, absurd, self-stultifying things that one so often finds oneself doing.' (Huxley, 1962)

---

[9] Johnson (1993) provides an extensive discussion of how moral reasoning is in many ways aesthetic in nature.

(A) *Jinverness Jidlewood presented to his psychiatrist with a history of having been abused as a child, and as having ongoing significant difficulties in interpersonal relationships. His relationship with therapists had similarly been characterized by a great deal of conflict; he often felt abused by therapists, and indeed in one case the psychotherapy did sound inappropriately harsh. Multiple trials of medications had failed to improve his low self-esteem and distrust of others. However, Jinverness had recently read Peter Kramer's book, and had reached the conclusion that Prozac was different, this was an ideal medication that would, he was certain, save his life.*

(B) *Kaley Kawalsky had been in insight-oriented psychotherapy for several years, and felt that she had gained a great deal. On the other hand, she suffered from a continuous sense of anhedonia. Although she herself did not meet the official criteria for a diagnosis of depression, several members of her family had suffered from this condition, and had responded well to fluoxetine. After reading a book about advances in the neurobiology of depression, Kaley decided that it was worth a trial of this medication. She discussed it with her therapist, and concluded that even if it failed, at least she would have tried all the options at her disposal.*

In his volume *Listening to Prozac*, Kramer described the effects of serotonin reuptake inhibitors in a series of patients who were in psychotherapy with him (Kramer, 1997). He noted that not only did symptoms of major depression improve, but that in some cases patients also experienced a fundamental change in the way they felt about life, viewed the world, and interacted with people. He therefore put forward the concept of "cosmetic psychopharmacology" – the potential use of psychotropics by people to improve relatively minor mood problems or to enhance temperament, analogous to the use of cosmetic surgery to enhance physical form. The value of enhancement therapies has been debated at length in the areas of genetic engineering and reproductive technologies.[10] It has also increasingly occupied authors interested in

---

[10] A range of authors have contributed to this literature (Anderson, 1989; Bayertz, 1994; Bostrom, 2007; Buchanan *et al.*, 2000; Budinger & Budinger, 2006; Daniels, 1994; Davis, 2001; Deane-Drummond & Scott, 2006; Fletcher, 1974; Fox, 2007; Fukuyama, 2002;

cosmetic surgery, endocrinology, sports medicine, and psychiatry.[11] An ongoing debate about the value of biotechnology and technology in general takes an often analogous form (Lightman et al., 2003; McKibben, 2003; Reiser, 1978; Rifkin, 1998; Shrader-Frechette & Westra, 1997; Stivers, 2004).

A classical view of medicine has tended to focus on disease rather than on physical or mental well-being. One reason for this may be the difficulty in finding consensus on what might constitute a decrease in well-being and in reliably measuring subtle forms of decreased well-being. There are also, however, ethical arguments for making a distinction between doctoring (treating dysfunction) and schmoctering (focusing on enhancement) and avoiding the latter (Parens, 1998b). Some authors (Daniels, 1994; Sabin & Daniels, 1994) argue on the basis of the principles of distributive justice that society need only provide resources for the former.[12] Others (bioconservatives[13]) argue that when

Garreau, 2005; Gehring, 2004; Glover, 1984; Habermas, 2003; Harris, 1992, 2007; Hattingh, 1992; Jonas 1974; Jones, 2005; Kitcher, 1996; Kurzweil, 2005; McGee, 1997; Mehlman, 2003; Murray, 2007; Naam, 2005; Nuffield Council on Bioethics, 2002; O'Donovan, 1984; O'Neill, 1985; Raymond, 1993; Reiss & Straughan, 1996; Resnik et al., 1999; Resnik & Vorhaus, 2006; Rifken, 1983; Robertson, 1994; Sandel, 2007; Silver, 1998; Stock, 2002; Stock & Campbell, 2000; Wailoo & Pemberton, 2006; Walters et al., 1997).

[11] A range of authors have contributed to this literature (Allen & Fost, 1990; Bolt & Mul, 2001; Bolt et al., 2002; Brown, 1984; Caplan, 2003; Caplan & Elliott, 2004; Charlton, 2003; Chatterjee, 2006; Davis, 1995a; DeGrazia, 2005; Diller, 1996; Elliott, 2003; Elliott & Chambers, 2004; Engelhardt, 1990; Ewing & Rosenbaum, 1994; Farah et al., 2004; Farah & Wolpe, 2004; Fox Keller, 1995; Fuchs, 2006; Glannon, 2006a; Gordijn, 2006; Hall, 2003; Hawthorne, 2007; Helmchen, 2005; Jacobson, 2000; Juengst, 2002; Kamm, 2005; Lock, 1993; Miah, 2004; Moreno, 2006a; Murray et al., 1984; Parens, 1998a, 1998b, 2006; Pellegrino, 2004; Perring, 1997b; Rees & Rose, 2004; Restak, 2003; Rose, 2002; Rothman & Rothman, 2003; Schwartz, 1991; Seaman, 2003; Tånnsjö & Tamburrini, 2000; Weisberger, 1995; Whitehouse et al., 1997; Wijsbek, 2000; Wolpe, 2002).

[12] Although one set of objections against enhancement has emphasized their costs (whether in terms of side effects or in terms of costs of equal access), these apply to both enhancements and treatments, and so are not a focus of the conceptual debate here. Instead, the focus here is mainly on the values associated with using enhancements (e.g. concerns about undermining natural order and eroding personal responsibility, or enforcing dubious norms and engendering psychological inauthenticity). Nevertheless, in a world where billions have little access to health care, but where some spend billions on baldness remedies, the costs of treatments–enhancements deserve to be a crucial consideration in our moral reasoning about their use (Mwase, 2005).

[13] I first came across this term in Jones (2006). There is a long history in Catholic thought of determining the "proper" functions of biological processes or organs of the body; for

medicine focuses on enhancement, it risks upsetting the natural order of things (Kass, 1985, 1995; President's Council on Bioethics, 2003). In the USA, the President's Council on Bioethics has argued that "[T]he naturalness of means matters. It lies not in the fact that the assisting drugs or devices are artefacts, but in the danger of violating or deforming the nature of human agency . . . biotechnology interventions act directly on the human body and mind to bring about their effects on a passive subject" (President's Council on Bioethics, 2003).

From a critical perspective, enhancement technologies, ranging from cosmetic surgery to cosmetic psychopharmacology, reinforce particular social constructions and values. The extension of medicine to include enhancement technologies is consistent with its role in decreasing social deviance, and is problematic insofar as it focuses on pathology and ignores resilience, overemphasizes technology and dehumanizes people, and ignores our overall physical, psychological, and spiritual well-being. Some psychotherapies may be useful in fostering self-knowledge and even self-transcendence (Cloninger, 2004), and some psychotropics (e.g. substances) may be of interest insofar as they allow an interrogation and deconstruction of "reality". However, just as cosmetic surgery reinforces particular social values (for example, equating women's looks with their value), so cosmetic psychopharmacology acts primarily as a conservative force, promoting inauthenticity and interfering with self-understanding (Crossley, 2003; Elliott, 2003; Murray, 2007; Rose, 1998a, 2007). As Murray (2007), for example, writes

Medicine is now the problem of the self; and medicine, we are told is the necessary solution to the problem – a problem that this medical discourse has in fact secretly produced and systematically obscured . . . the modern self remains constrained by a medical morality: I am morally remiss, my life is a life unworthy of living if I fail to submit to medical examinations, to doctors' and psychiatrists' recommendations.

Williams (1985) compares hyper-traditional societies, where there has been no exposure to contrasting views, with our modern world, where there is increasing exposure to a range of opinions. In a hyper-traditional

example, an emphasis on the procreative function of sexual intercourse is used to argue against the use of contraceptives (Blackford, 2006).

society, there may be little reflexive thought on where the boundaries of treatment should lie: the natural order of things is obvious. But since the dawn of the modern world, the lines between doctoring and schmoctoring have been open to debate, and ever-shifting. Following the approach of this volume, and of the previous section, an integrative perspective would be wary of any attempt to find a universal rule that differentiated between treatment and enhancement, or conversely, that rejected any possibility of a reasonable decision about where this line should be drawn. Again, the argument can be made that for any particular individual, conceptual and empirical work can help determine what the best intervention is, at any particular point in time. Still, although advances in biotechnology may be useful for a specific individual, the practices that they bring into play may also come with important costs.

As noted briefly in the introduction, there is a tension in Western society between values of self-improvement and self-creation, which would encourage people to use novel technologies including medical enhancement, and values around tradition and nature and about true self-discovery which argue that such changes are not authentic (Elliott, 2003; Parens, 1998b). In Huxley's "Island", the moksha-medicine suggests the possibility of using medication to enhance authenticity, but in his *Brave New World* soma serves to illustrate how psychopharmacological enhancement can be dehumanizing (Schermer, 2007). Given the emphasis that we place on effort in assigning responsibility for achievement, many view enhancement as representing diminished agency on the part of the person whose achievement is enhanced. However, Sandel, a member of the President's Council, counter-argues that both enhancement technologies, and also particularly high-pressure kinds of parenting (or "hyperparenting"), represent not so much a loss of agency, but rather hyperagency – an aspiration to remake nature, including human nature (Sandel, 2004). Mastery over nature, and self-improvement, have obvious benefits. But there is also the risk that viewing our talents solely as achievements for which we are responsible leads to hubris about ourselves (we are self-made and self-sufficient rather than merely fortunate), and a lack of solidarity with others less fortunate (who are deserving of their fate rather than merely unfortunate; Sandel, 2004).

What do the data from cognitive–affective science say? Earlier we used cognitive–affective data to argue that although the boundaries between disorder and normality are porous, our theory and value-based decisions about where to draw these lines can be reasonable ones. We also pointed out that although there were porous boundaries between psychotropics, nutrients, and substances, reasonable demarcations could be drawn. Similarly, if data emerge to show that particular interventions once considered "enhancements" are better understood as "treatments", these may appropriately move away from the domain of "schmoctering" and into that of "doctoring". Conversely, based on considered debate, we ought to be able to conclude that various medical interventions to help "normalize" people (for example, providing psychotherapy to turn gay people straight) should be scrapped. As Parens writes, "As one side emphasizes our obligation to remember that life is a gift and that we need to learn to let things be, the other emphasizes our obligation to transform that gift and to exhibit our creativity"(Parens, 2005).

Johnson has argued persuasively that moral reasoning is a special case of general (cognitive–affective) reasoning, and therefore must rely not so much on algorithmic rules as on the use of embodied metaphors. He notes that a moral tradition dating back to Plato, and including Descartes,[14] Kant and Rawls, makes a division between our bodies with their needs and passions, and a realm of freedom and reasons. However, moral rules do not exist as abstract entities; instead, moral reasoning is embodied in our brain-minds and in our social practices. It is precisely when our concepts of what is natural are challenged, for example, by new technologies, that the question of which metaphor to apply becomes particularly crucial.[15] Thus, in the case of cosmetic psychopharmacology (and other new technologies), we are left with

---

[14] Throughout the volume, Descartes has been criticized. This is somewhat unfair; it has been argued that his view of embodiment did more to permit the achievements of modern medicine than could any particular scientific theory, as it opened up the very possibility of a scientific medicine. Furthermore, he noted that feelings such as pain demonstrate that the mind is closely united with the body (Leder, 1984).

[15] Earlier, we noted that drugs can sometimes transform self-understanding. Johnson, following Dewey and Merleau-Ponty, notes that moral deliberation is also an activity of critical self-reflection and self-formation (Johnson, 1993).

the question of whether the MEDICAL metaphor of self-treatment (typically applied when some kind of unnatural breakdown occurs) or the MORAL metaphor of self-discovery (typically applied to every-day or apparently natural life), or a combination of the two, is more appropriate.[16] Life often presents us with conflicting moral solutions that cannot be hierarchically ordered by any universal principle. Those using psychotropics may find themselves using different metaphors at different times (Litton, 2005; Singh, 2005). Indeed, in medical prac-tice in general, and in cosmetic psychopharmacology in particular, the right balance between over-use and under-use of medical metaphors remains a matter of judgement.

Routine vaccination and fluoride supplementation are paradigmatic of health-care interventions that are undertaken in healthy children to strengthen them (rather than to treat a disorder), and that are now cor-rectly viewed as good doctoring. Similarly, folic acid is added to food to prevent neural tube defects in newborns, and vitamin supplemen-tation is recommended in healthy adults (Willett & Stampfer, 2001). Although the benefits of such practices have, on balance, been enor-mous, there have been significant costs for particular individuals (for example, those who have serious adverse reactions to vaccination). As interventions for high cholesterol and high blood pressure have been introduced, and become cheaper, so our cut-points for deciding who to treat have become less and less conservative. In the past it has been argued that antidepressants are only useful in those with major depres-sion, but there is now evidence that minor disorders are accompanied by significant disability (Kessler *et al.*, 2003) and also respond to these agents (Judd *et al.*, 2004). The risk–benefit of such interventions can be calculated using statistical measures such as numbers needed to treat and numbers needed to harm.

Although the analysis here has focused on disorder, analogous consi-derations would argue that no essentialist definition of health is possible, and its boundaries must be decided as reasonably as possible. The con-struct of "well-being" is often a component of our cognitive–affective

---

[16] In this context it is interesting to note the debate over whether bioethics should be a discipline of medicine or of philosophy.

maps for decision-making and moral judgements (Lakoff & Johnson, 1999), and may be more relevant to considering "enhancements" rather than "treatments". Given that humans do have some design flaws, and given advances in pharmaceuticals and psychotropics, it is not unlikely that more and more of these agents will be appropriately prescribed to more and more people for the purposes of well-being (Charlton, 2003; Chatterjee, 2006; Hall, 2003). It is not at all clear that there is any a priori ethical reason for rejecting a shift from a hyper-traditional view of doctoring, and moving to one that allows the employment of biotechnological advances to improve well-being (Caplan, 2003). Arguments that such advances threaten the natural order, for example, may simply reflect culture-specific views about what sort of conditions are needed for a good life (Blackford, 2006).[17] Indeed, political philosophers may disagree on whether a particular heritable disposition is a "natural primary good" (i.e. is valued across a range of diverse lives; Buchanan *et al.*, 2000; Fox, 2007),[18] and on the extent to which enhancement technologies should be regulated by the state (Resnik *et al.*, 1999; Stock, 2002). Nevertheless, even in the case of genetic engineering, many have defended a place for enhancement technologies in a society that allows its members to pursue well-being (Agar, 2004; Nozick, 1977; Rawls, 1971).[19]

---

[17] Hume (1739) emphasized that concepts of virtue could not be based on the "natural". Mill (1998) elaborated such distinctions further. Wittgenstein noted, "If you believe that our concepts are the right ones, the ones suited to intelligent human beings . . . then imagine certain general facts of nature different from the way they are, and concept structures different from our own will appear *natural* to you" (Wittgenstein, 1980). More recent authors have further argued that our ideas about what is natural reflect culture-specific views about the basic background conditions to human choice (Holland, 2003; Norman, 1996); explaining why such ideas are ordinarily viewed using the MORAL metaphor. However, we do not have to assume that apparently natural ways of doing things are incapable of improvement (Singer, 1993), and in a pluralistic society with changing background conditions (due to changing technology) what counts as an improvement may differ from individual to individual (Blackford, 2006).

[18] This idea draws on Rawls's concept of social primary goods (Rawls, 1971).

[19] The case of vaccination demonstrates how some prophylactic and promotive technologies may come to be seen as the responsibility of the state, albeit a contested responsibility (Bayer & Colgrove, 2002) where there is disagreement about the appropriateness of a MEDICAL versus MORAL approach.

On the other hand, there may be important costs associated with this kind of extension of doctoring. Given how well humans have been designed by evolution, the difficulties facing innovative science (Nightingale & Martin, 2004), and the high placebo response in those who suffer only mild impairment, it is hard to generate data showing that interventions to improve physical or psychological well-being are in fact effective and cost-effective. A growing empirical literature on happiness and well-being (Haidt, 2006) supports the view that gaining achievement at the cost of social connectedness is ultimately experienced as disadvantageous. Furthermore, raising expectations about the existence and value of enhancement technologies may be one of the reasons for the so-called "paradox of health" in contemporary societies; where populations that are in fact well, but also well-informed about pathology, complain more about disorder than unwell but uninformed groups (Barsky, 2005). Thus, the employment of biotechnological advances to improve well-being may at times be bad doctoring.

Earlier, we discussed the case of Abigail; she initially did not think of herself as having a disorder, but then after treatment came to a different conclusion. Conversely, however, there may well be cases where people inappropriately perceive themselves as requiring enhancement.[20] In a competitive society, for example, there may be an exaggeration of the extent to which cosmetic surgery or medication can give people an advantage. The pharmaceutical, alternative, and indigenous medicines industries and the media may play a particularly important role in encouraging the use of "lifestyle" surgeries and medications. Women and minorities may be particularly important targets (Davis, 1995a; Russell *et al.*, 1992). While it may be too far a reach to argue that advertisements about cosmetic surgery force women to undergo surgery, it certainly seems reasonable to argue that more varied ideals of beauty should be offered by society, that more rigorous evaluation of the motives of those wanting cosmetic surgery should be done, that more

---

[20] The term "critical interests" has been used to describe interests where satisfaction of interests would make a person's life genuinely better, and where a person would be genuinely mistaken if they did not recognize these interests (Dworkin, 1993; Nelson, 1995).

information should be given about the pros and cons of surgery, and that more knowledge about alternative approaches should be made available (Bolt *et al.*, 2002).

Neither evolutionary theory nor blanket ethical principles provide sufficient guidance for deciding on whether or not to medically intervene. A good example of this is the Dutch experiment with cosmetic surgery, which attempted to provide clinicians with rules such as "when a women looks 10 years beyond her age, surgery is permissible", and failed (Parens, 1998b). Suffering is a particularly important consideration in such decisions (Bolt *et al.*, 2002), but even here there are complexities, for example in determining the extent and appropriateness of suffering (and certainly not everyone who is distressed by imagined ugliness should receive cosmetic surgery (Phillips *et al.*, 1993)). In typical cases there is little debate; we can readily agree that plastic surgery to restore a normal appearance to a child who has suffered a severe facial burn is good doctoring, that using plastic surgery for an abused woman who believes that a changed appearance will stop her husband physically abusing her is bad doctoring, and that plastic surgery for a person who would like to look more like a favoured celebrity is schmoctering. In more atypical medical cases, however, an individualized clinical decision is required.

Similar considerations apply to the use of psychotropics. There is general agreement that prescribing psychotropics for depression is useful (see earlier section), that providing psychotropics to an abused woman in order to take away the pain in her current abusive relationship without supporting attempts to change or discontinue the relationship is bad doctoring (see the case of Jinverness above, where there may be over-optimism about the value of medication), and that using steroids with terrible side effects to enhance athletic performance is bad schmoctering. On the other hand, in some cases it would seem good judgement to try an "enhancement" in the hope that it would in fact serve as a useful "treatment" (e.g. as in the case of Kaley, a person with a strong family history of affective disorder, a genotype consistent with response to SSRI, and the wish to see if his low-grade mood improves on the medication). This position is consistent with a realist view that emphasizes an individualist approach to clinical decision-making, and that is neither overly optimistic nor unduly pessimistic about biotechnological advances.[21]

Just as the media cannot be held wholly responsible for modern ideals of beauty, so the pharmaceutical industry cannot be said to have entirely manufactured our concepts of either psychiatric disorder or mental fitness.[22] On the other hand, just as it is important to interrogate media constructs of beauty and to offer alternatives, so it is crucial to assess the extent to which the claims of the pharmaceutical, alternative, and indigenous medicines industries and other promoters of psychotropics go beyond the relevant science, and to offer a range of alternatives to those who may understandably want to use these agents to change their lives for the better. Psychopharmacology has the potential to liberate us by reducing the limits imposed on us by disorder, but to imprison us by imposing societal demands (Schwartz, 1991). In weighing up alternatives, it is certainly important to remember the excesses of past marketing campaigns (Angell, 2004; Degrandpre, 2006; Healy, 2004; McHenry, 2006; Moynihan & Smith, 2002; Smith, 1991; Starcevic, 2002; Szasz, 2001; Valenstein, 1998), and the overoptimism of researchers and clinicians about novel breakthroughs in psychopharmacology (van Praag, 1998). At the same time, and for particular

---

[21] Clinicians think about optimism and pessimism primarily in the context of prognosis. However, in the context of a debate about morality, one is reminded here of Strawson's contrast between pessimists who hold that deterministic causal explanations weaken concepts of responsibility and moral obligation, optimists who try to argue against this view, and Strawson's own attempt to reach a compatabilist position which is able to ground our moral concepts (Strawson, 1974). Flanagan also attempts an integrative approach to mind and morality, taking a naturalist approach and defending optimism (Flanagan, 2007). In discussing the future of biotechnology, Garreau contrasts a "Heaven Scenario", a "Hell Scenario", and a "Prevail Scenario" – a future in which technological crises are met with human resilience (Garreau, 2005). In putting forward an evolutionary perspective on modern culture, Humphrey compares "natural man" and "artificial man", and describes their possible interaction in terms of a civil war, a creative alliance, or a perfidious conspiracy – where we have to face the best and worse of modern civilization (Humphrey, 1999).

[22] There are circular interactions here; cultural norms encourage technologies, and technologies in turn reinforce cultural norms. In rarer cases, there is also more explicit coercion; for example, cosmetic surgery may be required for success in certain professions, and use of psychotropics to enhance performance in the military raises the possibility that this could be insisted upon.

individuals, at particular times, there is no reason to remain completely closed to the possibility that a specific psychotropic will turn out to be remarkably helpful. Good clinical practice invariably involves the kind of equipoise that comes from successfully balancing the perennial tensions described in this volume between the objective and subjective, explanation and understanding, and conflicting values.

Kaley's family history reminds us that a crucial area of advance in cognitive–affective science is human genomics. We now know that specific genetic variants, in interaction with particular environments, determine set-points in various neuronal circuits (Caspi & Moffitt, 2006; Mattay *et al.*, 2003; Pezawas *et al.*, 2005). We can no longer infer that all people experience pain or anxiety in the same way. Similarly, for particular individuals, certain psychotropics may be useful; people with the val–val polymorphism of the catechol-O-methyltransferase (COMT) gene are characterized by lower prefrontal dopamine levels and worse performance on working memory tasks, and may do well on certain medications – whereas people with the met–met COMT polymorphism have higher prefrontal dopamine levels and better performance, and may respond less well to the same agents (Stein, Newman, Savitz & Ramesar, 2006). On the basis of existing cognitive–affective science, it is possible to predict that in the future, physicians and psychopharmacologists will obtain detailed profiling of patients' genetic variants, and offer an individualized battery of medications and psychotropics (Buchanan *et al.*, 2002; Rothstein, 2003; van Delden *et al.*, 2004). There is the possibility that this will be done not merely to reduce conditions such as social anxiety and impulsivity, but also to increase well-being and enhance cognition.

On the other hand, it is important to emphasize the complexity of our genes and their interactions (Kendler, 2006), the unintended consequences of medication use, and the difficulties of coming up with elixirs that can outdo our evolutionary design (Jones, 2006; Nebert *et al.*, 2003; Nesse & Williams, 1994). An intervention that acts on only a few receptor targets may ultimately affect multiple processes in unpredictable ways. Just like the earlier "clinical gaze" (Foucault, 1973), so the more recent "molecular gaze" (Murray, 2007; Rose, 1998a) has its limitations. Indeed, despite much back-slapping about the value of current psychopharmacology, there has also been a great deal of exaggeration (van Praag, 1998). It is notable that currently available medications all work via only a few mechanisms, reflecting how difficult it is to make real breakthroughs in our pharmacopoeia. Similarly, current medications act on a fairly narrow range of phenomena (primarily mood and anxiety), and are relatively unhelpful for changing a range of other traits that may play a role in determining well-being (e.g. empathy). Again, to date, it is not yet clear whether available agents are better than, say, caffeine or exercise as cognitive enhancers. Thus, despite the already widespread use of psychotropics to improve well-being and enhance cognition, only time will tell how valuable for humans the field of cosmetic psychopharmacology will ultimately be.

The SSRIs deserve particular mention, as they have been key to this debate since the work of Kramer. It should be emphasized that, to date, there are relatively few empirical data on the use of psychotropics such as SSRIs in healthy volunteers. It is interesting that some controlled research demonstrates subtle changes in emotional processing and social behaviour in normals, sometimes outside of the awareness of subjects (Harmer *et al.*, 2004; Knutson *et al.*, 1998; Tse & Bond, 2002). Nevertheless, closer examination of such phenomena, as well as of the use of SSRIs in those with more significant symptomatology (even if it did not meet criteria for "major depression" or similar disorders), would be necessary to determine whether or not it was worthwhile. Currently there is insufficient evidence to argue that administration of an SSRI to healthy subjects results in increased well-being (Rego, 2005). Conversely, there is some evidence that SSRIs can flip predisposed people into a hypomanic state. However, this is an issue for further empirical work. Nutraceuticals, such as caffeine, and psychostimulant medications are widely used to enhance attention and memory, but again the evidence base to support the value of newer psychotropics as cognitive enhancers is currently sparse (Dekkers & Rikkert, 2007; Hall, 2003).

The difficulty of predicting response also applies to the particular case. Earlier, we gave the example of someone who decided that medication was a good/authentic choice only after starting it. Indeed, authenticity is not a static construct; Firlik (1991) and subsequent commentators (Elliott, 1999) provide a thought-provoking case of a woman who was against the artificial prolongation of life prior to suffering from dementia, but who can be seen as authentically in favour of artificial life support given her demented state. This is reminiscent of the earlier discussion, drawing from Parfit (1984), on personal identity; people are not fixed and immutable essences, they are more like clubs than like tables. In the absence of knowledge of pharmacogenetic predictors of response, and likely even if these were available, the ultimate value of a particular psychotropic for a patient may be difficult to predict until after it has been prescribed.

In summary, a classical approach to ethics in general, and to bioethics in particular, attempts to find moral rules for particular situations. In contrast, a critical approach argues that values inhere in our ways of life, and that ethics cannot be algorithmized. An integrative approach would argue that yes, values inhere in our way of life, but, first, these are closely related to our human nature – many would agree that pain is bad – and, second, they can be reasonably (i.e. cognitive–affectively) debated against the backdrop of particular circumstances (there are particular contexts in which pain may in fact be a reasonable choice). We cannot always reach universal conclusions about the nature of humans in general, or even the value of psychotropics (good or bad) in a specific patient. In the more subtle cases of cosmetic psychopharmacology a lack of ethical convergence is reinforced by a relative absence of empirical data. Nevertheless, in particular instances we can reach reasonable decisions – some lives are better than others. Relevant considerations for moral reasoning–imagining[23] about enhancements include both the potential value of stoic acceptance of life's fate (including imperfections and ageing, day-to-day distress, and idiosyncracies in personality), as well as the potential value of attempts to change the hand one is dealt (whether by virtue of pharmacotherapy, psychotherapy, or non-medical means). Some would argue that there can even be progress in moral reasoning (Bhaskar, 1979; MacIntyre, 1981).[24]

---

[23] To emphasize the importance of affect in reasoning, including moral reasoning, and drawing on Johnson's ideas about the importance of moral imagination, I use the double-barrel term reasoning–imagining here.

[24] A further, more controversial claim, is that there are "moral facts" (Casebeer, 2003; Dancy, 1993; McDowell, 1998).

The approach here is compatible with a growing interest in the field of neuroethics, with an emphasis on the value of empirical research in bioethics (Borry *et al.*, 2004), and with scientific work indicating that complex decision-making and moral judgements involve our cognitive–affective maps, which are in turn based on sensorimotor-affective neuronal circuitry and the way this allows interaction with the world.[25] It is notable that such work suggests that ethical concepts are learned by first understanding prototypical exemplars (Churchland, 2002; Stich, 2003), that moral reasoning involves both cognitive and affective processes and brain regions (Goldman, 1993a; Greene & Haidt, 2002), and that it becomes increasingly sophisticated during development (Kagan, 2006; Kohlberg, 1981). Further work by cognitive psychologists, linguists, neuroscientists, anthropologists, developmental and evolutionary scientists, and others are likely to lead to additional insights into the cognitive–affective bases of moral judgement (Stich, 1993). At the same time, the approach taken here has emphasized that human nature is sufficiently complex that debate about it will continue into the foreseeable future, and that even a detailed knowledge of the psychobiological basis of morality may encourage a diversity of values rather than a convergence in ethical thinking. Decisions about whether or not to use psychotropics are likely to remain controversial and given the relative complexity and difficulty of such decisions, this is certainly appropriate.

[25] Work relevant to this assertion has been undertaken by a range of authors (Churchland, 1998; de Waal *et al.*, 2006; Farah, 2005; Gibbard, 1990a; Goldman, 1993a; Greene & Haidt, 2002; Greene *et al.*, 2001; Hauser, 2006; Illes, 2006; Johnson, 1993; Joyce, 2006; Katz, 2001; Marcus, 2002; May *et al.*, 1996; Panksepp, 1998; Tancredi, 2005). Although "neuroethics" is a relatively new field, some of its concepts have early roots. Consider, for example, Aristotle's ideas about considering various exemplars to train oneself in moral reasoning, and Darwin's work "On the moral sense" (Goldman, 1993a).

7

Conclusion

The possibility of a naturalistic approach to the philosophy of psychopharmacology

Throughout this volume, we have begun by contrasting a classical approach (often referencing the viewpoint of one or other philosopher within the linguistic–analytic tradition) with various critiques of such an approach (often referencing the viewpoint of one or other continental philosopher). Then, rather than attempting to resolve this debate on its own philosophical terms, we have asked whether an integrative approach that uses some constructs drawn from each, and that is consistent with a realist philosophy, can be supported by data from contemporary cognitive-affective science. It has been suggested that such data generally reinforce a view that the mind-brain is embodied; sensorimotor and affective neuronal circuitry allows humans to interact with their physical and social world, and this in turn leads to the development of basic-level and abstract cognitive-affective maps (or metaphors) for understanding the world. These data support particular ways of approaching conceptual, explanatory and ethical questions in general, and issues in psychopharmacology in particular.

Is this the right way to do philosophy? It is certainly not one that would be widely accepted. Nevertheless, in my immediate defence, I would say that there is an important tradition in which philosophy is intended to be panoramic in scope, considering and integrating theories across disciplines and sciences. In ancient Greece, philosophy, or the "love of wisdom" covered a broad spectrum of questions. An early edition, however, divided Aristotle's corpus into the "Physica" (i.e. nature), which addressed natural philosophy, and the "Metaphysica" (i.e. the book after the Physica), where he addressed a series of more general questions and where he used the term "first philosophy". A formal split between natural philosophy (science) and philosophy is a relatively recent one, was not at all endorsed by Aristotle, and has been criticized by those interested in emphasizing that the subject matter of philosophy and of science is continuous.[1] Thornton, for example, has characterized philosophy of psychiatry as continuous with self-conscious psychiatry (Thornton, 2007).

Still, even if the subject matter of philosophy and of science is continuous, they may be very different endeavours, with quite different methods. Russell, a key philosopher in the classical tradition, argued that philosophy gives way to science only when conceptual issues have been sufficiently clarified that they can be empirically investigated (Russell, 1912). Similarly, the logical positivists and Wittgenstein emphasized the importance of dissolving meaningless philosophical questions. In this view, philosophy (which determines whether concepts make sense) plays a crucial role in assisting the sciences (which determines whether hypotheses make sense). In contrast, there are those who are more sceptical about the methods of science or philosophy. Philosophy may be useful insofar as it allows a more sceptical and critical view of science than science has of itself (Habermas, 1985). Philosophy may also be valuable in allowing reflection on possible solutions to profound questions, although the aim of solving such deep problems may be a futile one (McGinn, 1993). Thus, both the classical and critical views see philosophy and science as rather different fields of academic work.

On the other hand, many have argued that philosophy must increasingly address scientific data. For James and Jaspers, who contributed to philosophy and psychology, delineating the bonds between philosophy and science is a crucial task. As Merleau-Ponty writes, "From the

---

[1] As Piaget (1972b) put it, philosophy occupies itself with the study of knowledge as a whole, while science occupies itself with specific questions. Or, philosophy tends towards the study of being *qua* being, and science towards the knowledge of specific beings.

interrogation of science, philosophy stands to gain an encounter with certain articulations of being which otherwise it would find very difficult to uncover" (Merleau-Ponty, 1963a). An approach which emphasizes the value of scientific data has perhaps already won the battle for questions about the ultimate nature of matter (ontology), where philosophy in the absence of physics is no longer acceptable (Churchland, 2002). Furthermore, this view seems increasingly relevant to questions about explanation (epistemology), where an empirical epistemology (or neurophilosophy) now seems more and more desirable (Changeux, 2004; Quine, 1969). Finally, as noted briefly in the previous chapter, there is growing interest in the possibility that scientific data can also shed light on questions about moral judgement (ethics), so leading to an integration of science with ethics (or neuroethics) (Marcus, 2002).[2] It might also be argued that instead of using language solely as an analytic probe, philosophy could benefit by focusing on data that emerge from the science of linguistics.

One view which keeps philosophy and science as somewhat different endeavours, but which also emphasizes their continuities, is that philosophy, like science, is comprised of hypotheses. Locke viewed philosophy as removing impediments to knowledge, as an "underlabourer" to those who produced science (Locke, 1694). Bhaskar similarly views philosophy as conceptual science (Bhaskar, 1979), arguing that philosophy can serve to underpin or bootstrap empirical work.[3] This view is perhaps consistent with the idea that philosophy is one of the cognitive-affective sciences; its methods are more conceptual than empirical. Much contemporary philosophical writing is certainly naturalist in that it entails a view of humans as part of nature; a naturalistic view of ethics, for

---

[2] Dewey (1960) wrote that "the need for constant revision and expansion of moral knowledge is one great reason why there is no gulf between non-moral knowledge from that which is truly moral. At any moment concepts which once seemed to belong exclusively to the biological or psychological realm may assume moral import".

[3] Piaget asks, "does there exist an objective technique, that is to say, universally valid for the whole of knowledge?" And consistent with the position taken in the current volume, he answers, "Clearly there is none which would unite all thinkers: the concept of knowledge is still (and perhaps always will be) a matter of provisional synthesis, a synthesis which is in part subjective because it is in fact dominated by value judgments which are not universally applicable" (Piaget, 1972b).

example, may be contrasted with a supernaturalist view, and implies a focus on understanding ethics in worldly terms, rather than in terms of God or another transcendental authority (Grayling, 2004; Parfit, 1984; Williams, 1985). This kind of naturalistic approach to philosophy is again consistent with that taken in this volume, and would be accepted by many in the field.

Throughout this volume, when faced with complex classical and critical perspectives, we have asked the question of what the cognitive-affective data say. We have repeatedly argued that such data emphasize that human categories are not simply essentialist, but at the same time are not merely relativistic. Is there any evidence that science and philosophy themselves are human categories which cannot be defined using necessary and sufficient terms, but yet are not wholly subjective? Addressing this question in full falls outside the remit of this volume. Nevertheless, it is notable that efforts to define either the scientific or the philosophical method in an essentialist or algorithmic way remain incomplete. In particular, defining what counts as evidence remains a matter that is not straightforward; there is no "view from nowhere" (Nagel, 1989) from which such decisions can be made, instead they seem to require good judgement (for example, about conflicting scientific and philosophical virtues).

Indeed, questions about key constructs for science and philosophy, whether raised in the classic tradition (e.g. attempts by ancient philosophers and by Hume to define the nature of causation), or in the critical tradition (e.g. attempts to delineate human understanding and the space of reason), remain difficult to answer. Constructs such as "cause" may rather need to be understood in terms of prototypic exemplars, which are then extended to cover other phenomena (Johnson, 2003; Lakoff & Johnson, 1999; Piaget, 1972a). Churchland argues, for example, that scientists can agree on what counts as a prototypic explanation, but a range of more atypical exemplars may result in disagreement. Thus, good scientists use a mixture of conceptual thinking, empirical data and scientific values to make judgements about when to shift paradigms or change classifications. Analogously, Johnson (1993) has argued that the concept of morality is itself a radical category. Again, good clinicians use a mixture of conceptual thinking, empirical data and scientific values to make judgements about when to use the medical model and offer treatment.

But how do scientific and philosophical reasoning differ from everyday reasoning then? From one perspective on the cognitive-affective capacities of the brain-mind (Duchaine *et al.*, 2001), it could be argued that there is no privileged a priori approach to truth; instead, day-to-day cognition, science, and philosophy all involve living in the world, developing hypotheses, and modifying these based on experience. Pragmatists such as Peirce (1992) have suggested that there is no ultimate foundation to knowledge (scientific or philosophical); there is nothing that beats observing, experimenting, and analysing – using our brain-minds to re-examine our assumptions and revise them where necessary. At the same time, as our theoretical concepts become more sophisticated, and as our empirical database (including cognitive-affective data) increases, so our philosophical–scientific concepts become sharper and our explanations become more powerful (Churchland, 2002; Johnson, 1993; Lakoff & Johnson, 1999).

In this view, then, both scientific and philosophical reasoning, like other kinds of cognitive-affective processes and products, although not simply reducible to a set of formal and "objective" algorithms, have the potential to go beyond that which is merely "subjective" or relativistic. Like science, philosophical reasoning involves aspects that are both transitive (it is based within a social context) and intransitive (it is about the world; Bhaskar, 1978; Winch, 1970). It involves schemas which are on the one hand based in brain-mind, and on the other moulded by the participation of the brain-mind in the world. A naturalist approach to philosophy is consistent with scientific realism in general (Bhaskar, 1978) and embodied realism in particular (Lakoff & Johnson, 1999). It is also consistent with views that it is useful for philosophy to pay very close attention to scientific data (Churchland, 2002; Lakoff & Johnson, 1999), that philosophical and scientific hypotheses and explanations can themselves be the subject of useful empirical investigation (Carruthers *et al.*, 2002; Dunbar & Blanchette, 2001; Feist, 2006; Giere, 1988; Merton, 1973; Thagard, 1993, 2000), and that scientific realism is a conceptual hypothesis that helps to explain the success of science (Putnam, 1984).

We began the volume by emphasizing that any attempt to include a whole range of thinkers under a simple rubric (such as "classical" or "critical") must fail, and the aim of many of the contrasts drawn was to attempt to show some family resemblances, rather than to stake out necessary and sufficient criteria for belonging to the divergent schools of thought represented by the contrasting approaches to various philosophical questions posed here. We have gone on to suggest that cognitive-affective science holds that prototypes and metaphors are useful not only in understanding our day-to-day context, but also lie at the heart of our most sophisticated scientific and philosophical constructs. The categories of "classical" and "critical" themselves seem to reflect everyday mappings of crucial differences between notions of objective-disease/explanatory-cause/medical-treatment versus subjective-illness/understanding-reason/moral-acceptance; between choosing a MEDICAL and a MORAL metaphor. It is comforting that there is a certain consistency to the approach here; although little attempt was made to address directly the classical and critical approaches in their own conceptual terms, the strategy of relying on the relevant data from cognitive-affective science is compatible with a view that is sceptical of formal definitions of constructs, and also with the idea of using philosophical constructs as bootstraps to help conceptualize data and to reach valid explanations of the world.

Arguments that the approach here is consistent with a range of other work in philosophy, and also self-consistent, are perhaps not as pertinent, however, if the current volume does not take its premise of attempting to do conceptual science seriously. Has the work here made a contribution to its particular focus, namely the philosophy of psychiatry in general, and the philosophy of psychopharmacology in particular? Can it help provide a foundation for good clinical practice? I would begin by pointing out that in many ways this is a relatively undeveloped area of work. The psychiatrist and philosopher Karl Jaspers was perhaps the first to provide a rigorous philosophical analysis of the foundations of psychiatry, but this intersection requires further development. As Elliott (1999) argues, many philosophers have seen the problems raised by medicine and psychiatry as boring diversions, or as something altogether different from philosophy. However, with the introduction of new medical technologies, including psychotropics, new and important questions press for resolution.

After Jaspers, a range of thinkers considered the philosophical foundations of psychoanalysis, and defended psychiatry from the attacks of anti-psychiatry (Clare, 1967; Reznek, 1991; Roth & Kroll, 1986; Wing, 1978). During the further development of psychiatry and neuroscience, significant contributions continued to be made to developing the conceptual basis for psychiatric and clinical psychology practice and research, and to outlining the intersections between philosophy, psychopathology, and neuroscience.[4] The current volume contributes by demonstrating that psychopharmacology is a useful area for such work; it is valuable in addressing a range of conceptual issues (e.g. integrating facts and values in clinical nosology), explanatory issues (e.g. using explanation and understanding in the clinical practice), and ethical issues (e.g. balancing the appreciation of nature with a willingness to change it) that lie at the heart of the philosophy of psychiatry, and that are crucial for clinical practice.

A key conceptual issue in the volume was the nature of disorder in general. We argued that disorder cannot be understood in essentialist terms, but rather that disorder was a socially constructed category that was theory-bound and value-laden. We also argued, however, that our categories of disorder are not merely arbitrary or relativistic, but rather that typical disorders reflect universal biologically based concerns, and that decisions about whether to treat (pun intended) more atypical conditions as exemplars of disorder can be made in a reasonable way. Good nosology is based on well-considered judgements about concepts, data,

---

[4] A range of authors have contributed to developing the conceptual basis for psychiatric and clinical psychology practice and research (Bolton, 2008; Bolt & Hill, 1996; Brendel, 2006; Colby & Spar, 1983; Culver & Gert, 1982; Fulford *et al.*, 2003, 2006; Ghaemi, 2003; Gillett, 1999; Graham & Stephens, 1994; Griffiths, 1995; Hacking, 1998; Havens, 2004; Hundert, 1989; Kandel, 1998; Kendler, 2005; Kopelman, 1992; McHugh & Slawey, 1988; Miller, 1992; Radden, 2004; Sadler *et al.*, 1994; Schramme & Thome, 2004; Svensson, 1990; Tengland, 2001; Thornton, 2007a; Tyrer & Steinberg, 2005; Valentine, 1982; Wiggins & Schwartz, 1991; Zachar, 2000), and to outlining the intersections between philosophy, psychopathology, and neuroscience (Bechtel *et al.*, 2001; Bennett & Hacker, 2003; Bickle, 2003; Brook & Akins, 2005; Churchland, 2002; Illes, 2002, 2006; Marcus, 2002; Mishara, 2007).

and values. Psychiatric intervention is based on scientific knowledge, but its arts and practices also aim at the alleviation of human suffering. Thus, this volume falls within the Hippocratic tradition's emphasis on medicine as a science that engages with the complex realities of the human condition, and with the emphasis in the Hippocratic oath on practising with both skill and judgement (Gillett, 2006).[5]

Additional conceptual issues revolved around differentiating different kinds of psychotropic agents, addressing the nature of emotion, and considering various concepts of the self. Once again we took an approach that essentialist definitions of complex biological and psychiatric phenomena were unlikely to be found, but that it was nevertheless possible to defend a stance that was not entirely relativistic or subjective. Again, we argued that a realist position, which allowed for a scientific understanding of the structures and mechanisms of the world, including the embodiment of emotion and the self in the brain-mind and its interactions with the world, is supported by the cognitive-affective data in general, and by those from psychopharmacology in particular. Brain-minds are built on a constantly changing psychobiological foundation, and can be altered in powerful and unpredictable ways by nutrients, substances, nutraceuticals, and pharmaceuticals. For an individual patient, good clinical psychopharmacological practice requires an understanding not only of disease, but also of illness.

A number of explanatory issues were addressed, including the question of how best to explain pharmacotherapy and psychotherapy, how best to account for placebo responses, and the role of both proximal and distal (evolutionary) explanations. We argued that a functionalist account of the mind was not useful in explaining psychopharmacological phenomena. To understand how a psychotherapy changes the brain, or how the placebo effect is a crucial component of response to medication, or how a range of other conscious and unconscious cognitive-affective processes occur, we need a more complex model of

---

[5] Ghaemi has emphasized that Hippocrates took a cautious view towards medication, given that nature is the source of healing, and the job of the physician is to aid nature in the process of healing (Ghaemi, 2006). However, others have emphasized a view that the Hippocratic tradition involves finding moderation in the balance between opposite tendencies.

the brain-mind that provides explanations of symbols and their grounding, and of context and its brain-mind embodiment. Psychopharmacological phenomena are a useful tool-with-which-to-think about the links between explanation and understanding, mechanism and meaning, the sciences and the humanities, in psychology in general, and in biological psychiatry in particular.

In terms of ethical questions, we again attempted to move beyond classical and critical approaches, and to argue for an integrated position that psychopharmacology should not be viewed with unrealistic optimism nor with undue pessimism. Although there has not been a great deal of conceptual analysis in this area, some of those who have addressed the field of psychopharmacology appear to have suffered from psychotropic hedonism and from being overly optimistic about the future, others from pharmacological Calvinism and being overly pessimistic (Fukuyama, 2002; Klerman, 1972; van Praag, 1998). While we may not be able to reach complete ethical convergence about the value of modern psychotropics, in particular instances we can reach reasonable decisions for particular patients – some lives are better than others. Questions in psychopharmacology are a useful tool for addressing the broader philosophical debate on biotechnology in general; the view here may usefully be extended into other, structurally related, debates. Indeed, it is perhaps precisely when there are advances in science, when our concepts of the natural are challenged and where there is a need to bridge neuroscience and the person, that questions of which metaphor to apply become particularly interesting, and where practical questions can invigorate philosophy (Toulmin, 1982).

In summary, the hypotheses put forward here are useful insofar as they provide some conceptual progress towards laying out a path to the important goal of a better clinical psychopharmacology. We have offered a view of psychiatry and psychopharmacology that is naturalist insofar as it is based in the sciences, focused on the self and its disorders as embodied in the brain-mind and in social interactions, and employing relevant explanations (incorporating mechanisms and meanings, nature–nurture and their interaction, and proximal and distal variables). At the same time, we have aimed for a humanistic and non-reductionistic naturalism (Flanagan, 2007; Strawson, 1985); psychiatry and psychopharmacology must aim to engage fully with the complexities of the human condition, and to improve the lives of its patients. Psychiatric disorders comprise a large portion of the global burden of disease, and there are ongoing efforts to find effective and cost-effective treatments. Nevertheless, psychiatry has been accused of being either brainless or mindless (Eisenberg, 1995), with conceptual underpinnings that are often simplistic or dualist (Bolton & Hill, 1996). This volume hopefully makes a contribution by providing a more sophisticated account that integrates a range of perennial conceptual tensions in the field (objectivity/subjectivity, explanation/understanding, absolutism/relativism), and so assists the important goal of putting psychiatry and psychopharmacology on firmer footing.

References

Agar, N. (2004). *Liberal Eugenics: In Defense of Human Enhancement.* Oxford: Blackwell.

Ainslie, G. (2001). *Breakdown of Will.* Cambridge: Cambridge University Press.

Alderson, P. (1990). *Choosing for Children: Parent's Consent to Surgery.* Oxford: Oxford University Press.

Allen, D. B. & Fost, N. C. (1990). Growth hormone therapy for short stature: panacea or Pandora's Box? *Journal of Pediatrics*, **117**, 16–21.

American Psychiatric Association. (1994). *Diagnostic and Statistical Manual of Mental Disorders*, 4th edn. Washington, DC: American Psychiatric Press.

Anderson, W. F. (1989). Human gene therapy: why draw a line? *Journal of Medicine and Philosophy*, **14**, 681–9.

Angell, M. (2004). *The Truth About the Drug Companies: How They Deceive Us and What To Do About It.* New York, NY: Random House.

Arbib, M. A. & Fellous, J.-M. (2004). Emotions: from brain to robot. *Trends in Cognitive Science*, **8**, 554–61.

Aristotle. (1980). *Nichomachean Ethics.* Oxford: Oxford University Press.

Aristotle. (1984). *The Rhetoric and the Poetics of Aristotle.* New York, NY: McGraw-Hill.

Armstrong, D. M. & Malcolm, N. (1984). *Consciousness and Causality.* Oxford: Basil Blackwell.

Atkins, K. (2005). *Self and Subjectivity.* Malden, MA: Blackwell Publishing.

Ayer, A. J. (1936). *Language, Truth, and Logic.* London: Victor Gollancz.

Baier, A. (1985). *Postures of the Mind.* Minnesota, MN: University of Minnesota Press.

Ballenger, J. C., Davidson, J. A., Lecrubier, Y., *et al.* (1998). Consensus statement on social anxiety disorder from the international consensus group on depression and anxiety. *Journal of Clinical Psychiatry*, **59**, 54–60.

Barnes, B. (1974). *Scientific Knowledge and Sociological Theory*. London: Routledge.

Baron-Cohen, S. (1997). *The Maladapted Mind: Classic Readings in Evolutionary Psychopathology*. Hove, East Sussex: Psychology Press.

Barris, J. (1990). *God and Plastic Surgery: Marx, Nietzsche, Freud, and the Obvious*. Brooklyn, NY: Autonomedia.

Barsky, A. (2005). The paradox of health. *New England Journal of Medicine*, **318**, 414–18.

Baumeister, R. F., Bratslavsky, E., Finkenauer, C. & Vohs, K. D. (2001). Bad is stronger than good. *Review of General Psychology*, **5**, 323–70.

Baxter, L. R., Schwartz, J. M., Bergman, K. S., *et al.* (1992). Caudate glucose metabolic rate changes with both drug and behavior therapy for OCD. *Archives of General Psychiatry*, **49**, 681–9.

Bayer, R. & Colgrove, J. (2002). Science, politics and ideology in the campaign against environmental tobacco smoke. *American Journal of Public Health*, **92**, 949–54.

Bayertz, K. (1994). *GenEthics: Technological Intervention in Human Reproduction as a Philosophical Problem*. Cambridge: Cambridge University Press.

Beauchamp, T. L. & Childress, J. F. (2001). *Principles of Biomedical Ethics*, 5th edn. Oxford: Oxford University Press.

Bechtel, W., Mandik, P., Mundale, J. & Stufflebeam, R. S. (2001). *Philosophy and the Neurosciences: A Reader*. Oxford: Oxford University Press.

Ben-Ze'ev, A. (2000). *The Subtlety of Emotions*. Cambridge, MA and London, UK: MIT Press.

Bendesky, A. & Sonabend, A. M. (2005). On Schlepfuss' path: the placebo response in human evolution. *Medical Hypotheses*, **64**, 414–16.

Bennett, M. R. & Hacker, P. M. S. (2003). *Philosophical Foundations of Neuroscience*. Malden, MA: Blackwell.

Bentall, R. P. (1992). A proposal to classify happiness as a psychiatric disorder. *Journal of Medical Ethics*, **18**, 94–8.

Berlin, B. & Kay, P. (1969). *Basic Color Terms: Their Universality and Evolution*. Berkeley, CA: University of California Press.

Berlin, I. (1980). *Against the Current: Essays in the History of Ideas.* New York, NY: Viking Press.

Bermúdez, J. L., Marcel, A. & Eilan, N. (1995). *The Body and the Self.* Cambridge, MA: MIT Press.

Bernstein, R. J. (1983). *Beyond Objectivism and Relativism.* Oxford: Basil Blackwell.

Berry, C. J. (1986). *Human Nature.* Atlantic Highlands, NJ: Humanities Press International.

Bertens, H. (1995). *The Idea of the Postmodern: A History.* London: Routledge.

Bhaskar, R. (1978). *A Realist Theory of Science,* 2nd edn. Brighton, Sussex: Harvester Press.

Bhaskar, R. (1979). *The Possibility of Naturalism.* Brighton, Sussex: Harvester Press.

Bhaskar, R. (1986). *Scientific Realism & Human Emancipation.* London: Verso.

Bickle, J. (2003). *Philosophy and Neuroscience: A Ruthlessly Reductive Account.* Boston, MA: Kluwer Academic.

Bilder, R. M. & LeFever, F. F. (1998). Neuroscience of the mind on the centennial of Freud's project for a scientific psychology. *Annals of the New York Academy of Science,* **843**.

Blackburn, S. (1998). *Ruling Passions.* Oxford, Oxford University Press.

Blackford, R. (2006). Sinning against nature: the theory of background conditions. *Journal of Medical Ethics,* **32**, 629–34.

Blashfield, R., Sprock, J., Pinkston, K., *et al.* (1985). Exemplar prototypes of personality diagnoses. *Comprehensive Psychiatry,* **26**, 11–21.

Bloch, S. & Green, S. A. (2006). An ethical framework for psychiatry. *The British Journal of Psychiatry,* **188**, 7–12.

Block, N. J., Flanagan, O. J. & Güzeldere, G. (1997). *The Nature of Consciousness: Philosophical Debates.* Cambridge, MA: MIT Press.

Bloor, D. (1991). *Knowledge and Social Imagery.* London: Routledge.

Blum, L. (1980). *Friendship, Altruism, and Morality.* London: Routledge & Kegan Paul.

Bolt, I., Wijsbek, H., de Beaufort, I. & Hillhorst, M. (2002). Beauty and the Doctor: Moral Issues in Health Care with Regard to Appearance. Budel, Netherlands: Uitgeverij Damon.

Bolt, L. L. L. & Mul, D. (2001). Growth hormone in short children: beyond medicine? *Acta Paediatrica*, **90**, 69–73.

Bolton, D. (2000). Alternatives to disorder. *Philosophy, Psychiatry, & Psychology*, **7**, 141–53.

Bolton, D. (2004). Shifts in the philosophical foundations of psychiatry since Jaspers: implications for psychopathology and psychotherapy. *International Review of Psychiatry*, **16**, 184–9.

Bolton, D. (2008). *What is Mental Disorder? An Essay in Philosophy, Science, and Values.* Oxford: Oxford University Press.

Bolton, D. & Hill, J. (1996). *Mind, Meaning, and Mental Disorder: The Nature of Causal Explanation in Psychology and Psychiatry.* Oxford: Oxford University Press.

Boorse, C. (1975). On the distinction between disease and illness. *Philosophy and Public Affairs*, **5**, 49–68.

Boorse, C. (1976a). What a theory of mental health should be. *Journal of Theory Social Behaviour*, **6**, 61–84.

Boorse, C. (1976b). Wright on functions. *Journal of Theory of Social Behaviour*, **85**, 70–86.

Boorse, C. (1997). A rebuttal on health. In J. M. Humber & R. F. Almader (eds.) *What is Disease?* Totowa, NJ: Humana Press.

Borry, P., Schotsmans, P. & Dierickx, K. (2004). What is the role of empirical research in bioethical reflection and decision-making? An ethical analysis. *Medicine, Health Care and Philosophy*, **7**, 41–53.

Bosk, R. C. (1992). *All God's Mistakes: Genetic Counseling in a Pediatric Hospital.* Chicago, IL: Chicago University Press.

Bostrom, N. (2007). Human and genetic enhancements: a transhumanist perspective. *The Journal of Value Inquiry*, **37**, 493–506.

Bourdieu, P. (1998). *Practical Reason.* Stanford, CA: Stanford University Press.

Bowers, K. S. & Meichenbaum, D. (1984). *The Unconscious Reconsidered.* New York, NY: Wiley.

Bowlby, J. (1980). *Attachment and Loss*, Vol. 3. New York, NY: Basic Books.

Boyle, P. J. & Callahan, D. (1995). *What Price Mental Health? The Ethics and Politics of Setting Priorities.* Washington, DC: Georgetown University Press.

Bracken, P. & Thomas, P. (2005). *Postpsychiatry*. Oxford: Oxford University Press.

Bracken, P. J. (2003). Postmodernism and psychiatry. *Current Opinions in Psychiatry*, **16**, 673–7.

Braund, S. & Most, G. W. (2004). *Ancient Anger: Perspectives from Homer to Galen*. Cambridge: Cambridge University Press.

Breggin, P. (1993). *Toxic Psychiatry*. London: Fontana.

Brendel, D. H. (2006). *Healing Psychiatry: Bridging the Science/Humanism Divide*. Cambridge, MA: MIT Press.

Brentano, F. (1973). *Psychology From an Empirical Standpoint* (translated by A. Rancurello, D. B. Terrell & L. McAlister). New York, NY: Humanities Press.

Bridgman, P. W. (1927). *The Logic of Modern Physics*. New York, NY: Macmillan Press.

Brody, A. L., Saxena, S., Schwartz, J. M., *et al.* (1998). FDG-PET predictors of response to behavioral therapy and pharmacotherapy in obsessive compulsive disorder. *Psychiatry Research*, **84**, 1–6.

Brody, H. (1980). *Placebos and the Philosophy of Medicine: Clinical, Conceptual, and Ethical Issues*. Chicago: University of Chicago Press.

Brody, H. (2000). Three perspectives on the placebo response: expectancy, conditioning, and meaning. *Advances in Mind–Body Medicine*, **16**, 211–32.

Brook, A. & Akins, K. (2005). *Cognition and the Brain: The Philosophy and Neuroscience Movement*. Cambridge: Cambridge University Press.

Brown, W. M. (1984). Paternalism, drugs and the nature of sport. *Journal of the Philosophy of Sport*, **11**, 14–22.

Brülde, B. & Radovic, F. (2006). What is mental about mental disorder? *Philosophy, Psychiatry & Psychology*, **13**, 99–116.

Bruner, J. (1990). *Acts of Meaning*. Cambridge, MA: Harvard University Press.

Buchanan, A., Brock, D. W., Daniels, N. & Wikler, D. (2000). *From Chance to Choice: Genetics and Justice*. Cambridge: Cambridge University Press.

Buchanan, A., Califano, A., Kahn, J., McPherson, E., Robertson, J. & Brody, B. (2002). Pharmacogenetics: ethical issues and policy options. *Kennedy Institute of Ethics Journal*, **12**, 1–15.

Budinger, T. F. & Budinger, M. D. (2006). *Ethics of Emerging Technologies: Scientific Facts and Moral Challenges.* New York, NY: Wiley.

Bullard, A. (2002). From vastation to Prozac nation. *Transcultural Psychiatry,* **39**, 267–94.

Buller, D. J. (2005). *Adapting Minds: Evolutionary Psychology and the Persistent Quest for Human Nature.* Cambridge, MA: MIT Press.

Buss, D. M. (2000). The evolution of happiness. *American Psychologist,* **55**, 15–23.

Buss, D. M. (2005). *Handbook of Evolutionary Psychology.* New York, NY: John Wiley & Sons.

Buss, D. M., Haselton, M. G., Shackleford, T. K., Bleske, A. L. & Wakefield, J. C. (1998). Adaptations, exaptations, and spandrels. *American Psychologist,* **53**, 533–48.

Callahan, D. (2003). *What Price Better Health? Hazards of the Research Imperative.* Berkeley, CA: University of California Press.

Campbell, E. J. M., Scadding, J. G. & Roberts, R. S. (1979). The concept of disease. *British Medical Journal,* **2**, 757–62.

Campbell-Sills, L. & Stein, M. B. (2005). Justifying the diagnostic status of social phobia: a reply to Wakefield, Horwitz, and Schmitz. *Canadian Journal of Psychiatry,* **50**, 320–3.

Canguilhem, G. (1966). *The Normal and the Pathological.* New York, NY: Urzone.

Cannon, W. B. (1927). The James–Lange theory of emotion: a critical examination and an alternative theory. *American Journal of Psychology,* **39**, 106–24.

Cantor, N., Smith, E. E., French, R. D. & Mezzich, J. (1980). Psychiatric diagnosis as prototype categorization. *Journal of Abnormal Psychology,* **89**, 181–93.

Caplan, A. (2003). Is better best? *Scientific American,* **289**, 104–5.

Caplan, A. & Elliott, C. (2004). Is it ethical to use enhancement technologies to make us better than well? *PLoS Medicine,* **1**, 172–5.

Caplan, A. L. (1981). The 'Unnaturalness of aging' – A sickness unto death? In A. L. Caplan, H. T. Engelhardt Jr & J. J. McCartney eds. *Concepts of Health and Disease: An Interdisciplinary Perspective.* Reading, MA: Addison-Wesley, pp. 725–38.

Caplan, A. L., Engelhardt, H. T. J. & McCartney, J. J. (1981). *Concepts of Health and Disease: Interdisciplinary Perspectives.* Reading, MA: Addison-Wesley Publishing.

Carlsten, A., Waern, M., Ekedahl, A. & Ranstam, J. (2001). Antidepressant medication and suicide in Sweden. *Pharmacoepidemiology and Drug Safety,* **10**, 525–30.

Carruthers, P., Stich, S. & Siegal, M. (2002). *The Cognitive Basis of Science.* Cambridge: Cambridge University Press.

Carson, R. & Burns, C. (1997). *Philosophy of Medicine and Bioethics.* Dordrecht: Kluwer.

Cartwright, N. (2007). Are RCTs the gold standard? *BioSocieties,* **2**, 11–20.

Cartwright, S. A. (1981). Report of the diseases and physical peculiarities of the Negro race. In A. L. Caplan, H. T. Engelhardt Jr & J. J. McCartney, eds. *Concepts of Health and Disease: Interdisciplinary Perspectives.* Reading, MA: Addison-Wesley, pp. 305–26.

Casebeer, W. (2003). *Natural Ethical Facts: Evolution, Connectionism, and Moral Cognition.* Cambridge, MA: MIT Press.

Caspi, A. & Moffitt, T. E. (2006). Gene–environment interactions in psychiatry: joining forces with neuroscience. *Nature Reviews in Neuroscience,* **7**, 583–90.

Cavalli-Sforza, L. L. & Feldman, M. W. (1981). *Cultural Transmission and Evolution: A Quantitative Approach.* Princeton, NJ: Princeton University Press.

Chalmers, D. (1995). *The Conscious Mind: In Search of a Fundamental Theory.* New York, NY: Oxford University Press.

Chambers, T. (1999). *The Fiction of Bioethics: Cases as Literary Texts.* New York, NY: Routledge.

Changeux, J.-P. (2004). *The Physiology of Truth: Neuroscience and Human Knowledge.* Cambridge, MA: Harvard University Press.

Charlton, B. G. (2003). Palliative psychopharmacology: a putative speciality to optimize the subjective quality of life. *Quarterly Journal of Medicine,* **96**, 375–8.

Chatterjee, A. (2006). The promise and predicament of cosmetic neurology. *Journal of Medical Ethics,* **32**, 110–13.

Chisholm, D., Sanderson, K., Ayuso-Mateos, J. L. & Saxena, S. (2004). Reducing the global burden of depression: population-level analysis of intervention cost-effectiveness in 14 world regions. *British Journal of Psychiatry,* **164**, 393–403.

Churchland, P. (1995). *The Engine of Reason, the Seat of the Soul: A Philosophical Journey into the Brain.* Cambridge, MA: MIT Press.

Churchland, P. M. (1998). Toward a cognitive neurobiology of the moral virtues: moral reasoning. *Topoi,* **17**, 83–96.

Churchland, P. S. (2002). *Brain-Wise: Studies in Neurophilosophy.* Cambridge, MA: MIT Press.

Cilliers, P. (1998). *Complexity and Postmodernism: Understanding Complex Systems.* London: Routledge.

Clare, A. (1967). *Psychiatry in Dissent.* London: Tavistock Publications.

Clark, A. (1997). *Being There: Putting Brain, Body and World Together.* Cambridge, MA: MIT Press.

Clark, A. (2001). *Mindware: An Introduction to the Philosophy of Cognitive Science.* Oxford: Oxford University Press.

Clark, P. & Wright, C. (1988). *Mind, Psychoanalysis and Science.* Oxford: Blackwell.

Clark, T. W. (2007). *Encouraging Naturalism: A Worldview and Its Uses.* Somerville, MA: Center for Naturalism.

Cloninger, C. R. (1987). A systematic method for clinical descriptions and classification of personality variants. *Archives of General Psychiatry,* **44**, 573–88.

Cloninger, C. R. (2004). *Feeling Good: The Science of Well Being.* New York, NY: Oxford University Press.

Colby, K. M. & Spar, J. E. (1983). *The Fundamental Crisis in Psychiatry: Unreliability of Diagnosis.* Springfield, IL: Charles C. Thomas.

Cole-Turner, R. (1998). Do means matter? In E. Parens, ed. *Enhancing Human Traits: Ethical and Social Considerations.* Washington, DC: Georgetown University Press, pp. 151–61.

Collins, H. M. (1985). *Changing Order.* London: Sage.

Conrad, P. & Schneider, J. (1980). *Deviance and Medicalization: From Badness to Sickness.* St. Louis, MO: Mosby.

Cosmides, L. & Tooby, J. (1999). Toward an evolutionary taxonomy of treatable conditions. *Journal of Abnormal Psychology,* **108**, 453–64.

Cosmides, L. & Tooby, T. (2003). *What is Evolutionary Psychology? Explaining the New Science of Mind.* New Haven, CT: Yale University.

Coyne, J. C. & Marcus, S. C. (2006). Health disparities in care for depression possibly obscured by the clinical significance criterion. *American Journal of Psychiatry,* **163**, 1577–9.

Crick, F. & Koch, C. (2003). A framework for consciousness. *Nature Neuroscience*, **6**, 119–26.

Crossley, N. (2003). Prozac nation and the biochemical self. In S. Williams, L. Birke & G. Bendelow, eds. *Debating Biology: Sociological Reflections on Health, Medicine, and Society*. London: Routledge.

Culver, C. M. & Gert, B. (1982). *Philosophy in Medicine: Conceptual and Ethical Issues in Medicine and Psychiatry*. Oxford: Oxford University Press.

Damasio, A. (1999). *The Feeling of What Happens: Body and Emotion in the Making of Consciousness*. San Diego, CA: Harcourt Brace.

Damasio, A. (2003). *Looking for Spinoza: Joy, Sorrow, and the Feeling Brain*. San Diego, CA: Harcourt.

Damasio, A. R. (1994). *Descartes' Error: Emotion, Reason, and the Human Brain*. New York, NY: HarperCollins.

Damasio, A. R. (1996). The somatic marker hypothesis and the possible functions of the prefrontal cortex. *Philosophical Transactions of the Royal Society*, **351**, 1413–20.

Dancy, J. (1993). *Moral Reasons*. Oxford: Blackwell Publishers.

Daniels, N. (1994). The genome project, individual differences, and just health care. In T. F. Murphy & M. A. Lappe, eds. *Justice and the Human Genome Project*. Berkeley, CA: University of California Press.

Darwin, C. (1965). *The Expression of Emotion in Man and Animals*. Chicago, IL: Chicago University Press, p. 1872.

Davidson, D. (1984). *Inquiries into Truth and Interpretation*. Oxford: Oxford University Press.

Davidson, R. J. (2003). Seven sins in the study of emotion: correctives from affective neuroscience. *Brain and Cognition*, **52**, 129–32.

Davies, P. S. (2003). *Norms of Nature: Naturalism and the Nature of Functions*. Cambridge, MA: MIT Press.

Davis, D. (2001). *Genetic Dilemmas*. New York, NY: Routledge.

Davis, H. J. (2004). Dementia: sociological and philosophical constructions. *Social Science and Medicine*, **58**, 369–78.

Davis, K. (1995a). *Reshaping the Female Body: The Dilemma of Cosmetic Surgery*. New York, NY: Routledge.

Davis, L. J. (1995b). *Enforcing Normalcy: Disability, Deafness and the Body*. New York, NY: Verso.

de Beaufort, I., Bolt, I., Hilhorst, M. & Wijsbek, H. (2000). Beauty and the Doctor: Moral Issues in Health Care with Regard to Appearance: Final Report of a European Project. European Commission.

De Botton, A. (2001). *The Consolations of Philosophy*. London: Penguin Books.

de la Fuente-Fernandez, R., Ruth, T. J., Sossi, V., Schulzer, M., Calne, D. B. & Stoessl, A. J. (2001). Expectation and dopamine release: mechanism of the placebo effect in Parkinson's disease. *Science, 293*, 1164–6.

de la Fuente-Fernández, S. M. & Stoessl, A. J. (2004). Placebo mechanisms and reward circuitry: clues from Parkinson's disease. *Biological Psychiatry, 56*, 67–71.

de Sousa, R. (1987). *The Rationality of the Emotions*. Cambridge, MA: MIT Press.

de Spinoza, B. (1677). *Ethics: On the Origin and Nature of the Emotions*. Whitefish, MT: Kessinger Publishing [2004].

de Waal, F. B. M., Macedo, S., Ober, J. & Korsgaard, C. M. (2006). *Primates and Philosophers: How Morality Evolved*. Princeton, NJ: Princeton University Press.

Dean, W., Morgenthaler, J. & Fowkes, S. W. (1993). *Smart Drugs II – The Next Generation: New Drugs and Nutrients to Improve Your Memory and Increase Your Intelligence*. Menlo Park, CA: Health Freedom Publications.

Deane-Drummond, C. & Scott, P. (2006). *Future Perfect? God, Medicine and Human Identity*. London: T&T Clark.

Decety, J. & Sommerville, J. A. (2003). Shared representations between self and other: a social cognitive neuroscience view. *Trends in Cognitive Sciences, 7*, 527–33.

Degenaar, J. (1979). Some philosophical considerations on pain. *The Journal of the International Association for the Study of Pain, 7*, 281–304.

Degrandpre, R. (2006). *The Cult of Pharmacology*. Durham, NC: Duke University Press.

DeGrazia, D. (2005). Enhancement technologies and human identity. *Journal of Medicine and Philosophy,* **30**, 261–83.

Dekkers, W. & Rikkert, M. O. (2007). Memory enhancing drugs and Alzheimer's disease: enhancing the self or preventing the loss of it? *Medicine, Health Care and Philosophy,* **10**, 141–51.

Delancey, C. (2001). *Passionate Engines: What Emotions Reveal about Mind and Artificial Intelligence.* Oxford, Oxford University Press.

Delay, J. (2006). Psychopharmacology and psychiatry. *Presse Medicale,* **74**, 1151–6.

Deleuze, G. (1995). *Negotiations* (translated by M. Joughlin). New York, NY: Columbia University Press.

Deltito, J. A. & Stam, M. (1989). Psychopharmacological treatment of avoidant personality disorder. *Comprehensive Psychiatry,* **30**, 498–504.

Demyttenaere, K., Bruffaerts, R., Posada-Villa, J., *et al.* (2004). Prevalence, severity, and unmet need for treatment of mental disorders in the World Health Organization World Mental Health Surveys. *Journal of the American Medical Association,* **291**, 2581–90.

Dennett, D. (1987). *The Intentional Stance.* Cambridge, MA: MIT Press.

Dennett, D. C. (1991). *Consciousness Explained.* Boston, MA: Little, Brown & Co.

Dennett, D. C. (1995). *Darwin's Dangerous Idea: Evolution and the Meanings of Life.* New York, NY: Simon and Schuster.

Dennett, D. C. (2003). *Freedom Evolves.* London: Penguin.

Descartes, R. (1650). *The Passions of the Soul.* Indianapolis, IN: Hackett Publishing Company [1989].

Descartes, R. (1993). *Meditations on First Philosophy* (translated by D. A. Cress). Indianapolis, IN: Hackett.

DeVries, R. & Subedi, J. (1998). *Bioethics and Society: Constructing the Ethical Enterprise.* Upper Saddle River, NJ: Prentice Hall.

Dewey, J. (1960). *Theory of the Moral Life.* New York, NY: Holt, Rinehart, and Winston.

Di Blasi, Z., Kaptchuk, T. J., Weinman, J. & Kleijnen, J. (2002). Informing participants of allocation to placebo at trial closure: postal survey. *British Medical Journal,* **325**, 1329.

Diller, L. H. (1996). The run on Ritalin: attention deficit disorder and stimulant treatment in the 1990s. *Hastings Center Report,* **26**, 12–18.

Dilman, I. (1999). *Free Will: An Historical and Philosophical Introduction.* London: Routledge.

Dilthey, W. (1883). *Introduction to the Human Sciences* (translated by R. Makkreel & F. Rodi). Princeton, NJ: Princeton University Press [1989].

Dolan, R. J. (2002). Emotion, cognition, and behavior. *Science,* **298**, 1191–4.

Douglas, M. (1984). *Purity and Danger: An Analysis of Concepts of Pollution and Taboo.* London: Routledge.

Dowling, J. E. (2004). *The Great Brain Debate: Nature or Nurture.* Washington, DC: Joseph Henry Press.

Doyal, L. (1979). *The Political Economy of Health.* London: Pluto Press.

Dreyfus, H. L. (2005). Merleau-Ponty and recent cognitive science. In T. Carman & M. B. Hansen, eds. *The Cambridge Companion to Merleau-Ponty.* Cambridge: Cambridge University Press.

Duchaine, B., Cosmides, L. & Tooby, J. (2001). Evolutionary psychology and the brain. *Current Opinion in Neurobiology,* **11**, 225–30.

Duff, R. A. (1986). *Trials and Punishments.* Cambridge: Cambridge University Press.

Dumit, J. (2004). *Picturing Personhood: Brain Scans and Biomedical Identity.* Princeton, NJ: Princeton University Press.

Dunbar, K. & Blanchette, I. (2001). The *in vivo/in vitro* approach to cognition: the case of analogy. *Trends in Cognitive Science* **5**, 334–9.

Dworkin, R. (1993). *Life's Dominion.* New York, NY: Alfred A. Knopf.

Dworkin, R. W. (2006). *Artificial Happiness: The Dark Side of the New Happy Class.* New York, NY: Graf & Graf Publishers.

Eccles, J. C. (1994). *How the Self Controls Its Brain.* Berlin, Springer.

Edelman, G. M. (2003). Naturalizing consciousness: a theoretical framework. *Proceedings of the National Academy of Sciences USA,* **100**, 5520–4.

Ehrenreich, B. & English, B. (1973). *Complaints and Disorders: The Sexual Politics of Sickness.* Old Westbury, NY: The Feminist Press.

Eisenberg, L. (1995). The social construction of the human brain. *American Journal of Psychiatry,* **152**, 1563–75.

Eldridge, R. (1989). *On Moral Personhood: Philosophy, Literature, Criticism, and Self-understanding.* Chicago, IL: University of Chicago Press.

Ellenberger, H. F. (1970). *The Discovery of the Unconscious: The History and Evolution of Dynamic Psychiatry.* New York, NY: Basic Books.

Elliott, A. (2001). *Concepts of the Self.* London: Blackwell.

Elliott, C. (1996). *The Rules of Insanity: Moral Responsibility and the Mentally Ill.* Albany, NY: State University of New York Press.

Elliott, C. (1999). *A Philosophical Disease: Bioethics, Culture and Identity.* New York, NY: Routledge.

Elliott, C. (2003). *Better than Well: American Medicine Meets the American Dream.* New York, NY: Norton.

Elliott, C. (2007). Against happiness. *Medicine, Health Care and Philosophy,* **10**, 167–71.

Elliott, C. & Chambers, T. (2004). *Prozac as a Way of Life.* Chapel Hill, NC: University of North Carolina Press.

Elster, J. (1999a). *Alchemies of the Mind: Rationality and the Emotions.* Cambridge: Cambridge University Press.

Elster, J. (1999b). *Strong Feelings: Emotion, Addition and Human Behavior.* Cambridge, MA: MIT Press.

Emanuel, E. J. & Miller, F. K. (2001). The ethics of placebo-controlled trials – a middle ground. *New England Journal of Medicine,* **345**, 915–19.

Engel, G. L. (1977). The need for a new medical model: a challenge for biomedicine. *Science,* **196**, 129–36.

Engelhardt, H. T. (1990). Human nature technologically revisited. *Social Philosophy and Policy,* **8**, 180–91.

Engelhardt, H. T. & Spicker, S. F. (1977). Mental Health: Philosophical Perspectives: Proceedings of the Fourth Trans-Disciplinary Symposium on Philosophy and Medicine, held at Galveston: Tx. Dordrecht: D. Reidel.

Engelhardt, H. T. J. (1973). Psychotherapy as meta-ethics. *Psychiatry,* **36**, 440–5.

Engelhardt, H. T. J. (2000). *The Philosophy of Medicine: Framing the Field.* Dordrecht: Kluwer Academic Publishers.

Erchak, G. (1992). *The Anthropology of Self and Behavior.* New Brunswick, NJ: Rutgers University Press.

Erdelyi, M. H. (1985). *Psychoanalysis: Freud's Cognitive Psychology.* New York, NY: WH Freeman.

Evans, D. (2003). *Placebo: The Belief Effect.* New York, NY: HarperCollins.

Evans, D. & Cruse, P. (2004). *Emotion, Evolution, and Rationality.* Oxford: Oxford University Press.

Evans, J. H. (2002). *Playing God? Human Genetic Engineering and the Rationalization of Public Bioethical Debate.* Chicago, IL: Chicago University Press.

Ewing, S. E. & Rosenbaum, J. F. (1994). Phrenotropics: makeup for the mind? *Harvard Review of Psychiatry,* **2**, 49–51.

Farah, M. J. (2005). Neuroethics: the practical and the philosophical. *Trends in Cognitive Sciences,* **9**, 34–40.

Farah, M. J., Illes, R., Cook-Deegan, R., *et al.* (2004). Neurocognitive enhancement: what can we do? what should we do? *Nature Reviews Neuroscience,* **5**, 412–25.

Farah, M. J. & Wolpe, P. R. (2004). Monitoring and manipulating brain function: new neuroscience technologies and their ethical implications. *Hastings Center Report,* **34**, 35–45.

Farmer, P. (2003). *Pathologies of Power: Health, Human Rights, and the New War on the Poor.* Berkeley, CA: University of California Press.

Fawcett, J., Stein, D. J. & Jobson, K. O. (1999). *Textbook of Treatment Algorithms in Psychopharmacology.* Chichester: John Wiley & Sons.

Feinberg, T. E. (2001). *Altered Egos: How the Brain Creates the Self.* New York, NY: Oxford University Press.

Feinberg, T. E. & Keenan, J. P. (2005). *The Lost Self: Pathologies of the Brain and Identity.* New York, NY: Oxford University Press.

Feist, G. J. (2006). *The Psychology of Science and the Origins of the Scientific Mind.* New Haven, CT: Yale University Press.

Feyerabend, P. (1975). *Against Method.* Verso: London.

Firlik, A. (1991). Margo's logo. *Journal of the American Medical Association,* **265**, 201.

First, M. B., Pincus, H. A., Levine, J. B., Williams, J. B. W., Ustun, B. & Peele, R. (2004). Clinical utility as a criterion for revising psychiatric diagnoses. *American Journal of Psychiatry,* **161**, 946–54.

Flanagan, O. (1991). *Varieties of Moral Personality: Ethics and Psychological Realism.* Cambridge, MA: Harvard University Press.

Flanagan, O. (1998). *Self Expressions: Mind, Morals, and the Meaning of Life.* Oxford: Oxford University Press.

Flanagan, O. (2003). *The Problem of the Soul: Two Visions of Mind and How to Reconcile Them.* New York: Basic Books.

Flanagan, O. (2007). *The Really Hard Problem: Meaning in a Material World.* New York, NY: Bradford Books.

Fletcher, J. (1974). *The Ethics of Genetics Control: Ending Reproductive Roulette.* New York: Anchor Books.

Fletcher, J. (1975). The cognitive criterion of personhood. *Hastings Center Report,* **4**, 4–7.

Flew, A. (1973). *Crime or Disease?* New York, NY: Barnes and Noble.

Flower, R. (2004). Lifestyle drugs: pharmacology and the social agenda. *Trends in Pharmacological Sciences,* **25**, 182–5.

Fodor, J. A. (1975). *The Language of Thought.* New York, NY: Crowell.

Fodor, J. A. (1987). *Psychosemantics.* Cambridge, MA: MIT Press.

Fodor, J. A. (2000). *The Mind Doesn't Work that Way: The Scope and Limits of Computational Psychology.* Cambridge, MA: MIT Press.

Foot, P. (2003). *Natural Goodness.* Oxford: Oxford University Press.

Forte, R., Hoffman, A., Wasson, R. G., *et al.* (2000). *Entheogens and the Future of Religion.* The Council on Spiritual Practices, 2nd edn. Thousand Oaks, CA: Pine Forge Press.

Foucault, M. (1973). *The Birth of the Clinic.* London: Tavistock.

Fox Keller, E. (1995). *Refiguring Life: Metaphors of Twentieth-century Biology.* New York, NY: Columbia University Press.

Fox, D. (2007). The illiberality of 'liberal eugenics'. *Ratio,* **20**, 1–25.

Fox, R. C. & Swazey, J. P. (1992). *Spare Parts: Organ Replacement and American Society.* Oxford: Oxford University Press.

Frances, A. & Clarkin, J. F. (1981). No treatment as the prescription of choice. *Archives of General Psychiatry,* **38**, 542–5.

Frank, A. (1979). *Wounded Storyteller: Body, Illness and Ethics.* Chicago, IL: University of Chicago Press.

Frank, R. H. (1988). *Passions Within Reason: The Strategic Role of the Emotions.* New York, NY: Norton.

Freud, S. (1917). Mourning and melancholia. In *Standard Edition,* Vol. 14, 1957. London: Hogarth.

Freud, S. (1961). Civilization and its Discontents. In *Standard Edition,* Vol. 21, London: Hogarth Press, p. 66.

Fuchs, T. (2006). Ethical issues in neuroscience. *Current Opinion in Psychiatry,* **19**, 600–7.

Fukuyama, F. (2002). *Our Posthuman Future: Consequences of the Biotechnology Revolution.* New York, NY: Farrar Straus Giroux.

Fulford, K. W. (2002). Values in psychiatric diagnosis: executive summary of a report to the chair of the ICD-12/DSM-VI coordination task force (dateline 2010). *Psychopathology,* **35**, 132–8.

Fulford, K. W., Broome, W., Stanghellini, G. & Thornton, T. (2005). Looking with both eyes open: fact and value in psychiatric diagnosis? *World Psychiatry,* **4**, 78–86.

Fulford, K. W. M. (1989). *Moral Theory and Medical Practice.* Cambridge: Cambridge University Press.

Fulford, K. W. M. (1999). Nine variations and a coda on the theme of an evolutionary definition of dysfunction. *Journal of Abnormal Psychology,* **108**, 412–20.

Fulford, K. W. M. (2001). 'What is (mental) disease?': an open letter to Christopher Boorse. *Journal of Medical Ethics,* **27**, 80–5.

Fulford, K. W. M., Morris, K., Sadler, J. & Stanghellini, G. (2003). *Nature and Narrative.* Oxford: Oxford University Press.

Fulford, K. W. M., Thornton, T. & Graham, G. (2006). *Oxford Textbook of Philosophy and Psychiatry.* Oxford: Oxford University Press.

Furmark, T., Tillfors, M., Marteinsdottir, I., *et al.* (2002). Common changes in cerebral blood flow in patients with social phobia treated with citalopram or cognitive-behavioral therapy. *Archives of General Psychiatry,* **59**, 425–33.

Fusar-Poli, P. & Broome, M. R. (2006). Conceptual issues in psychiatric neuroimaging. *Current Opinion in Psychiatry,* **19**, 608–12.

Fux, M., Levine, J., Aviv, A., *et al.* (1996). Inositol treatment of obsessive–compulsive disorder. *American Journal of Psychiatry,* **153**, 1219–21.

Gadamer, H.-G. (1993). *The Enigma of Health: The Art of Healing in a Scientific Age.* Cambridge: Polity Press.

Gallagher, S. (2000). Philosophical conceptions of the self: implications for cognitive science. *Trends in Cognitive Sciences,* **4**, 14–21.

Gallagher, S. (2005). *How the Body Shapes the Mind.* Oxford: Oxford University Press.

Gardner, H. (1985). *The Mind's New Science: A History of the Cognitive Revolution.* New York, NY: Basic Books.

Gardner, J. (1978). *Moral Fiction.* New York, NY: Basic Books.

Garfield, S. F., Smith, F. J. & Francis, S.-A. (2003). The paradoxical role of antidepressant medication – returning to normal functioning while losing the sense of being normal. *Journal of Mental Health,* **12**, 521–35.

Garland, B. (2004). *Neuroscience and the Law: Brain, Mind, and the Scales of Justice.* New York, NY: Charles A. Dana Foundation.

Garreau, J. (2005). *Radical Evolution: The Promise and Peril of Enhancing Our Minds, Our Bodies – And What it Means to be Human.* New York, NY: Doubleday.

Gazzaniga, M. (1998). *The Mind's Past.* New York, NY: Basic Books.

Gehring, V. V. (2004). *Genetic Prospects: Essays on Biotechnology, Ethics, and Public Policy.* Lanham, MD: Rowman & Littlefield.

Gellner, E. (1985). *Relativism and the Social Sciences.* Cambridge: Cambridge University Press.

Gerard, M. S. & Higley, J. D. (2002). Evolutionary underpinnings of excessive alcohol consumption. *Addiction,* **97**, 415–25.

Ghaemi, N. (2003). *Concepts of Psychiatry.* Baltimore, MD: Johns Hopkins University Press.

Ghaemi, S. N. (2006). Hippocratic psychopharmacology for bipolar disorder – an expert's opinion. *Psychiatry,* **3**, June, 30–45.

Gibbard, A. (1990a). *Wise Choices, Apt Feelings.* Cambridge, MA: Harvard University Press.

Gibbard, A. (1990b). *Wise Choices, Apt Feelings: A Theory of Normative Judgment.* Cambridge, MA: Harvard University Press.

Gibbs, R. W. J. (2006). *Embodiment and Cognitive Science.* Cambridge: Cambridge University Press.

Gibson, J. J. (1977). The theory of affordances. In R. E. Shaw & J. Bransford, eds. *Perceiving, Acting, and Knowing.* Hillsdale, NJ: Erlbaum.

Giddens, A. (1984). *The Constitution of Society.* Berkeley, CA: University of California Press.

Giddens, A. (1991). *Modernity and Self-Identity: Self and Society in the Late Modern Age.* Stanford, CA: Stanford University Press.

Giere, R. N. (1988). *Explaining Science: A Cognitive Approach.* Chicago, IL: University of Chicago Press.

Gillett, G. (1999). *The Mind and its Discontents*. Oxford: Oxford University Press.

Gillett, G. (2006). Medical science, culture, and truth. *Philosophy, Ethics, and Humanities in Medicine,* **1**, 13.

Glannon, W. (2006a). *Bioethics and the Brain*. Oxford: Oxford University Press.

Glannon, W. (2006b). Psychopharmacology and memory. *Journal of Medical Ethics,* **32**, 74–8.

Glas, G. (2004). Philosophical aspects of neurobiological research on anxiety and anxiety disorders. *Current Opinion in Psychiatry,* **17**, 457–64.

Glover, J. (1970). *Responsibility*. London: Routledge and Kegan Paul.

Glover, J. (1984). *What Sort of People Should There Be?* New York, NY: Pelican Books.

Glover, J. (1988). *The Philosophy and Psychology of Personal Identity*. London: The Penguin Group.

Goldberg, A. (2007). *Moral Stealth: How "Correct Behavior" Insinuates Itself into Psychotherapeutic Practice*. Chicago, IL: University of Chicago Press.

Goldie, P. (2000). *The Emotions: A Philosophical Exploration*. Oxford: Oxford University Press.

Goldie, P. (2004). *On Personality*. London: Routledge.

Goldman, A. I. (1993a). Ethics and cognitive science. *Ethics,* **103**, 337–60.

Goldman, A. I. (1993b). *Readings in Philosophy and Cognitive Science*. Cambridge, MA: MIT Press.

Goleman, D. (1996). *Vital Lies Simple Truths: The Psychology of Self Deception*. New York, NY: Simon and Shuster.

Goodman, A. (1991). Organic unity theory: the mind–body problem revised. *American Journal of Psychiatry,* **148**, 553–63.

Gopnik, A., Meltzoff, A. N. & Kuhl, P. K. (1999). *The Scientist in the Crib*. New York, NY: Morrow.

Gordijn, B. (2006). *Medical Utopias: Ethical Observations*. Louvain, Paris and Dudley, MA: Peeters Publishers.

Gordon, R. (1987). *The Structure of Emotions: Investigations in Cognitive Psychology*. Cambridge: Cambridge University Press.

Gosling, J. C. (1965). *Pleasure and Desire.* Oxford: Oxford University Press.

Gould, S. J. (1991). Exaptation: a crucial tool for evolutionary psychology. *Journal of Social Issues,* **47**, 43–65.

Graham, G. (1990). Melancholic epistemology. *Synthese,* **82**, 399–422.

Graham, G. & Stephens, G. L. (1994). *Philosophical Psychopathology.* Cambridge, MA: The MIT Press.

Grayling, A. C. (2004). *What is Good?* London: Orion.

Greenberg, L. & Safran, J. (1991). *Emotion, Psychotherapy, and Change.* New York, NY: Guilford Press.

Greene, J. & Haidt, J. (2002). How (and where) does moral judgment work? *Trends in Cognitive Sciences,* **12**, 517–23.

Greene, J. D. & Cohen, J. D. (2004). For the law, neuroscience changes nothing and everything. *Philosophical Transactions of the Royal Society London,* **359**, 1775–85.

Greene, J. D., Sommerville, R. B., Nystrom, L. E., Darley, J. M. & Cohen, J. D. (2001). An fMRI investigation of emotional engagement in moral judgment. *Science,* **293**, 2105–8.

Greenhalgh, T. & Hurwitz, B. (1998). *Narrative Based Medicine: Dialogue and Discourse in Clinical Practice.* London: BMJ Books.

Greenspan, P. (1988). *Emotions and Reasons: An Inquiry into Emotional Justification.* New York: Routledge, Chapman and Hall.

Greenwood, J. D. (1991). *The Future of Folk Psychology: Intentionality and Cognitive Science.* Cambridge: Cambridge University Press.

Grene, M. & Depew, D. (2004). *The Philosophy of Biology: An Episodic History.* Cambridge: Cambridge University Press.

Griffiths, A. P. (1995). *Philosophy, Psychology, and Psychiatry.* Cambridge: Cambridge University Press.

Griffiths, P. (1997). *What Emotions Really Are: The Problem of Psychological Categories.* Chicago, IL: University of Chicago Press.

Griffiths, R. R., Richards, W. A., McCann, U. & Jesse, R. (2006). Psilocybin can occasion mystical-type experiences having substantial and sustained personal meaning and spiritual significance. *Psychopharmacology,* **187**, 268–83.

Grünbaum, A. (1985). *The Foundations of Psychoanalysis: A Philosophical Critique.* Berkeley, CA: University of California Press.

Guess, H. A., Kleinman, A., Kusek, J. W. & Engel, L. W. (2002). *The Science of the Placebo: Toward an Interdisciplinary Research Agenda.* London: BMJ Books.

Guze, S. B. (1989). Biological psychiatry: is there any other kind? *Psychological Medicine* **19**, 315–23.

Haack, S. (2003). *Defending Science – Within Reason.* Amherst, NY: Prometheus Books.

Haaga, D. A. & Beck, A. T. (1995). Perspectives on depressive realism: implications for cognitive theory of depression. *Behaviour Research and Therapy,* **33**, 41–8.

Habermas, J. (1971). *Knowledge and Human Interests* (translated by J. J. Shapiro). Boston, MA: Beacon Press.

Habermas, J. (1985). *Philosophical–Political Profiles.* Cambridge, MA: MIT Press.

Habermas, J. (2003). *The Future of Human Nature.* Cambridge: Polity Press.

Hacker, P. M. S. (2004). The conceptual framework for the investigation of emotions. *International Review of Psychiatry,* **16**, 199–208.

Hacking, I. (1998). *Mad Travelers: Reflection on the Reality of Transient Mental Illnesses.* Charlottesville, VA: University Press of Virginia.

Haidt, J. (2006). *The Happiness Hypothesis: Putting Ancient Wisdom to the Test of Modern Science.* New York, NY: Random House.

Haimes, E. (2002). What can the social sciences contribute to the study of ethics? Theoretical, empirical and substantive considerations. *Bioethics,* **16**, 89–113.

Hall, S. S. (2003). The quest for a smart pill. *Scientific American,* **289**, 54–65.

Hamann, S., Ely, T. D., Grafton, S. T. & Kilts, C. D. (1999). Amygdala activity related to enhanced memory for pleasant and aversive stimuli. *Nature Neuroscience,* **2**, 289–93.

Hamilton, J. A., Jensvold, M. & Rothblum, E. D. (1995). *Psychopharmacology from a Feminist Perspective.* Binghamton, NY: Haworth Press.

Hamilton, V., Bower, G. & Frijda, N. (1988). *Cognitive Perspectives on Emotion and Motivation.* Dordrecht: Kluwer.

Hampshire, S. (1983). *Morality and Conflict.* London: Basil Blackwell.

Hampshire, S. (2005). *Spinoza and Spinozism.* Oxford: Oxford University Press.

Hansen, J. & Maynes, J. (2005). Psychiatry, philosophy and the self. *Current Opinions in Psychiatry,* **18,** 649–52.

Hardy, G., Hardy, I. & Ball, P. A. (2003). Neutraceuticals – a pharmaceutical viewpoint: Part II. *Current Opinions in Clinical Nutrition and Metabolic Care,* **6,** 661–71.

Hare, R. M. (1952). *The Language of Morals.* Oxford: Oxford University Press.

Hare, R. M. (1963). *Freedom and Reason.* Oxford: Clarendon.

Hare, R. M. (1983). Medical ethics, can the moral philosopher help? In R. M. Hare, ed. *Essays on Bioethics.* Oxford: Clarendon Press.

Harman, G. & Thomson, J. J. (1996). Moral Relativism and Moral Objectivity. Oxford: Blackwell Publishers.

Harmer, C. J., Shelley, N. C., Cowen, P. J. & Goodwin, G. M. (2004). Increased positive versus negative affective perception and memory in healthy volunteers following selective serotonin and norepinephrine reuptake inhibition. *American Journal of Psychiatry,* **161,** 1256–63.

Harnad, S. (1989). Minds, machines, and Searle. *Journal of Theoretical and Experimental Artificial Intelligence,* **1,** 5–25.

Harnad, S. (1990). The symbol grounding problem. *Physica,* **42,** 335–46.

Harré, R. (1983). *Personal Being.* Oxford: Blackwell.

Harré, R. (1986a). *Varieties of Realism: A Rationale for the Natural Sciences.* Oxford: Basil Blackwell.

Harré, R. (1986b). *The Social Construction of Emotions.* Oxford: Blackwell.

Harré, R. & Gillett, G. (1994). *The Discursive Mind.* Thousand Oaks, CA: Sage Publications.

Harrington, A. (1999). *The Placebo Effect: An Interdisciplinary Collaboration.* Cambridge, MA: Harvard University Press.

Harris, J. (1987). QALYfying the value of life. *Journal of Medical Ethics,* **13,** 117–23.

Harris, J. (1992). *Wonderwoman and Superman: The Ethics of Human Biotechnology.* Oxford: Oxford University Press.

Harris, J. (2007). *Enhancing Evolution: The Ethical Case for Making Better People.* Princeton, NJ: Princeton University Press.

Harrison, B. (1979). *An Introduction to the Philosophy of Language.* London: McMillan.

Hart, H. L. A. (1968). *Punishment and Responsibility: Essays in the Philosophy of Law.* Oxford: Oxford University Press.

Harter, S. (1999). *The Construction of the Self: A Developmental Perspective.* New York, NY: The Guilford Press.

Hattingh, J. (1992). *Genetic Engineering in Ethical Perspective.* Stellenbosch: Unit for Bio-medical Ethics of the University of Stellenbosch.

Hatzimoysis, A. (2003). *Philosophy and the Emotions.* Cambridge: Cambridge University Press.

Hauser, M. D. (2006). *Moral Minds.* New York, NY: Ecco (HarperCollins).

Havens, L. L. (2004). *Psychiatric Movements: Approaches to the Mind.* Cambridge, MA: Harvard University Press.

Hawthorne, S. (2007). ADHD drugs: values that drive the debates and decisions. *Medicine, Health Care and Philosophy,* **10**, 129–40.

Healy, D. (2002). *The Creation of Psychopharmacology.* Cambridge, MA: Harvard University Press.

Healy, D. (2004). *Let Them Eat Prozac: The Unhealthy Relationship Between the Pharmaceutical Industry and Depression.* New York, NY: New York University Press.

Hedgecoe, A. M. (2004). Critical bioethics: beyond the social science critique of applied ethics. *Bioethics,* **18**, 120–43.

Heginbotham, C. (2000). *Philosophy, Psychiatry and Psychopathy: Personal Identity in Mental Disorder.* Aldershot: Ashgate Publishing Ltd.

Heidegger, M. (1962). *Being and Time.* New York, NY: Harper.

Heidegger, M. (1999). *The Question Concerning Technology. Basic Writings.* London: Routledge.

Helgason, T., Tomasson, H. & Zoega, T. (2004). Antidepressants and public health in Iceland. Time series analysis of national data. *British Journal of Psychiatry,* **184**, 157–62.

Helm, B. (2001). *Emotional Reason: Deliberation, Motivation, and the Nature of Value.* Cambridge: Cambridge University Press.

Helmchen, H. (2005). Forthcoming ethical issues in biological psychiatry. *World Journal of Biological Psychiatry,* **6S2**, 56–64.

Hempel, C. G. (1965). *Aspects of Scientific Explanation and Other Essays in the Philosophy of Science.* New York, NY: Free Press.

Henriques, J., Hollway, W., Urwin, C., Venn, C. & Walkerdine, V. (1984). *Changing the Subject: Psychology, Social Regulation and Subjectivity.* London and New York: Methuen.

Henry, M., Fishman, J. R., & Younger, S. J. (2007). Propranolol and the prevention of post-traumatic stress disorder: is it wrong to erase the "sting" of bad memories? *American Journal of Bioethics,* **7**, 12–20.

Hobson, J. A. (2001). *The Dream Drugstore: Chemically Altered States of Consciousness.* Cambridge, MA: MIT Press.

Hoffmaster, B. (2000). *Bioethics in a Social Context.* Philadelphia, PA: Temple University Press.

Holland, S. (2003). *Bioethics: A Philosophical Introduction.* Cambridge: Polity Press.

Holmes, D., Murray, S. J., Perron, A. & Rail, G. (2006). Deconstructing the evidence-based discourse in health sciences: truth, power, and fascism. *International Journal of Evidence-Based Healthcare,* **4**, 180–6.

Holmes, J. & Lindley, R. (1989). *The Values of Psychotherapy.* Oxford: Oxford University Press.

Homer (2006). *The Odyssey* (translated by R. Fagles). New York, NY: Penguin.

Hook, S. (1959). *Psychoanalysis, Scientific Method, and Philosophy.* New York, NY: New York University Press.

Horne, R., Graupner, L., Frost, S., Weinman, J., Wright, S. M. & Hankins, M. (2004). Medicine in a multi-cultural society: the effect of cultural background on beliefs about medications. *Social Science and Medicine,* **59**, 1307–13.

Horowitz, L. M., Post, D. L., French, R., *et al.* (1981). The prototype as a construct in abnormal psychology: 2. Clarifying disagreement in psychiatric judgments. *Journal of Abnormal Psychology,* **90**, 575–85.

Horwitz, A. V. & Wakefield, J. C. (2007). *The Loss of Sadness: How Psychiatry Transformed Normal Sorrow into Depressive Disorder.* New York: Oxford University Press.

Hrobjartsson, A. & Gotzsche, P. C. (2001). Is the placebo powerless? An analysis of clinical trails comparing placebo with no treatment. *New England Journal of Medicine,* **344**, 1594–602.

Hudson, J. I. & Pope, H. G. J. (1990). Affective spectrum disorder: does antidepressant response identify a family of disorders with a common pathophysiology? *American Journal of Psychiatry,* **147**, 552–64.

Hull, D. & Ruse, M. (2007). *The Cambridge Companion to the Philosophy of Biology*. Cambridge: Cambridge University Press.

Humber, J. M. & Almeder, F. (1997). *What is Disease?* Totowa, NJ: Humana Press.

Hume, D. (1739). *A Treatise of Human Nature*. London: Penguin Classics [1985].

Humphrey, N. (1999). *A History of the Mind: Evolution and the Birth of Consciousness*. Berlin: Springer.

Humphrey, N. (2002). *The Mind Made Flesh*. Oxford: Oxford University Press.

Hundert, E. (1989). *Philosophy, Psychiatry and Neuroscience: Three Approaches to the Mind*. Oxford: Oxford University Press.

Hurley, S. L. (1998). *Consciousness in Action*. Cambridge, MA: Harvard University Press.

Husak, D. N. (1992). *Drugs and Rights*. Cambridge: Cambridge University Press.

Hursthouse, R. (1999). *On Virtue Ethics*. Oxford: Clarendon Press.

Huxley, A. (1932). *Brave New World*. London: Chatto & Windus.

Huxley, A. (1954). *The Doors of Perception*. New York, NY: Harper.

Huxley, A. (1962). *Island*. New York, NY: HarperCollins Publishers.

Illes, J. (2002). Ethical challenges in advanced neuroimaging. Special issue. *Brain and Cognition,* **50**, 341–523.

Illes, J. (2006). *Neuroethics: Defining the Issues in Theory, Practice, and Policy*. Oxford: Oxford University Press.

Illich, I. (1977). *Limits to Medicine: Medical Nemesis: The Expropriation of Health*. New York, NY: Penguin Books.

IMS Health. (2002). IMS Drug Monitor. Antidepressants Vol. 2002. Available at: http://www.imshealth.com/ims/portal/front/articleC/ 0,2777,6025/3665_1005394,00.html.

Ingleby, D. (1981). *Critical Psychiatry: The Politics of Mental Health*. New York, NY: Penguin.

Jablensky, A. (2005). Boundaries of mental disorders. *Current Opinions in Psychiatry,* **18**, 653–8.

Jacobson, N. (2000). *Cleavage: Technology, Controversy, and the Ironies of the Man-Made Breast.* New Brunswick, NJ: Rutgers University Press.

James, W. (1884). What is an emotion? *Mind,* **9**, 188–205.

James, W. (1890). *The Principles of Psychology.* New York, NY: Henry Holt.

James, W. (1907). *Pragmatism.* Cambridge, MA: Harvard University Press [1979].

Jaspers, K. (1963). *General Psychopathology.* Chicago, IL: Chicago University Press.

Johnson, M. (1993). *Moral Imagination: Implications of Cognitive Science for Ethics.* Chicago, IL: University of Chicago Press.

Johnson, S. P. (2003). The nature of cognitive development. *Trends in Cognitive Sciences,* **7**, 102–4.

Johnston, P. (1989). *Wittgenstein and Moral Philosophy.* London: Macmillan.

Jonas, H. (1974). *Philosophical Essays from Ancient Creed to Technological Man.* Englewood Cliffs, NJ: Prentice Hall.

Jones, D. G. (2005). *Designers of the Future.* Oxford: Monarch.

Jones, D. G. (2006). Enhancement: are ethicists excessively influenced by baseless speculations? *Medical Humanities,* **32**, 77–81.

Jonsen, A. R. (2000). *A Short History of Medical Ethics.* New York and Oxford: Oxford University Press.

Jorm, A. F. (2000). Mental health literacy. Public knowledge and beliefs about mental disorders. *British Journal of Psychiatry,* **177**, 396–401.

Joyce, R. (2006). *The Evolution of Morality.* Cambridge, MA: MIT Press.

Judd, L. L., Rapoport, M. H., Yonkers, K. A., *et al.* (2004). Randomized, placebo-controlled trial of fluoxetine for acute treatment of minor depressive disorder. *American Journal of Psychiatry,* **161**, 1864–71.

Juengst, E. T. (2002). Growing pains: bioethical perspectives on growth hormone replacement research. *Journal of Anti-Aging Medicine,* **5**, 73–9.

Kadison, R. (2005). Getting an edge – use of stimulants and antidepressants in college. *New England Journal of Medicine,* **353**, 1089–91.

Kagan, J. (2006). *An Argument for Mind.* New Haven, CT: Yale University Press.

Kagan, J., Reznick, J. S. & Gibbons, J. (1988). Biological basis of childhood shyness. *Science*, **240**, 167–71.

Kahneman, D. & Tversky, A. (2000). *Choices, Values, and Frames*. New York, NY: Cambridge University Press.

Kamm, F. M. (2005). Is there a problem with enhancement? *American Journal of Bioethics*, **5**, 5–14.

Kandel, E. R. (1998). A new intellectual framework for psychiatry. *American Journal of Psychiatry*, **155**, 457–69.

Kane, R. (2001). *Free Will*. Oxford: Oxford University Press.

Kant, I. (1781). *Critique of Pure Reason* (translated by J. M. D. Meiklejohn). London: NuVision Publications [2005].

Kant, I. (1785). *Grounding for the Metaphysics of Morals* (translated by J. W. Ellington). Indianapolis, IN: Hackett.

Kant, I. (1977). *Prolegomena to Any Future Metaphysics* (translated by J. W. Ellington). Indianapolis, IN: Hackett.

Kass, L. (1985). *Towards a More Natural Science*. New York, NY: Free Press.

Kass, L. R. (1995). The end of courtship. *The Public Interest*, **126**, 39–63.

Katz, L. D. (2001). *Evolutionary Origins of Morality*. Bowling Green, OH: Imprint Academic.

Kay, P. & McDaniel, C. (1978). The linguistic significance of the meanings of basic color terms. *Language*, **54**, 610–46.

Keat, R. & Urry, J. (1982). *Social Theory as Science*, 2nd edn. London: Routledge and Kegan Paul.

Keenan, J. P., Gallup, G. G. & Falk, D. (2001). *The Face in the Mirror: How the Brain Creates the Self*. New York, NY: HarperCollins/Ecco.

Kendell, R. & Jablensky, A. (2003). Distinguishing between the validity and utility of psychiatric diagnosis. *American Journal of Psychiatry*, **160**, 4–12.

Kendell, R. E. (1975). The concept of disease and its implications for psychiatry. *British Journal of Psychiatry*, **127**, 305–15.

Kendler, K. S. (1990). Towards a scientific nosology: strengths and limitations. *Archives of General Psychiatry*, **47**, 969–73.

Kendler, K. S. (2001). A psychiatric dialogue on the mind–body problem. *American Journal of Psychiatry*, **158**, 989–1000.

Kendler, K. S. (2005). Toward a philosophical structure for psychiatry. *American Journal of Psychiatry*, **162**, 433–40.

Kendler, K. S. (2006). Reflections on the relationship between psychiatric genetics and psychiatric nosology. *American Journal of Psychiatry*, **163**, 1138–46.

Kenny, A. (1963). *Action, Emotion and the Will.* London: Routledge & Kegan Paul.

Kenny, A. J. P. (1969). Mental health in Plato's Republic. Proceedings of the Aristotelian Society, 3 December, 229–53.

Kessler, R. C. (2002). The categorical versus dimensional assessment controversy in the sociology of mental illness. *Journal of Health and Social Behavior*, **43**, 171–88.

Kessler, R. C., Merikangas, K. R., Berglund, P., Easton, W. W., Koretz, D. S. & Walters, M. S. (2003). Mild disorders should not be eliminated from the DSM-V. *Archives of General Psychiatry*, **60**, 1117–22.

Kierkegaard, S. (1981). *The Concept of Anxiety.* Princeton, NJ: Princeton University Press.

Kihlstrom, J. F. (1987). The cognitive unconscious. *Science*, **237**, 1145–51.

Kircher, T. & David, A. (2003). *The Self in Neuroscience and Psychiatry.* Cambridge: Cambridge University Press.

Kitcher, P. (1985). *Vaulting Ambition: Sociobiology and the Quest for Human Nature.* Cambridge, MA: MIT Press.

Kitcher, P. (1996). *The Lives to Come: The Genetic Revolution and Human Possibilities.* New York, NY: Simon and Schuster.

Klein, D. F. (1964). Delineation of two drug-responsive anxiety syndromes. *Psychopharmacologia*, **5**, 397–408.

Klein, D. F. (1978). A proposed definition of mental illness. In R. L. Spitzer & D. F. Klein, eds. *Critical Issues in Psychiatric Diagnosis.* New York, NY: Raven Press, pp. 41–71.

Klein, D. F. (1993). Clinical psychopharmacological practice: the need for a developing research base. *Archives of General Psychiatry*, **50**, 491–4.

Klein, D. F., Thase, M. E., Endicott, J., *et al.* (2002). Improving clinical trials: American Society of Clinical Psychopharmacology recommendations. *Archives of General Psychiatry*, **59**, 272–8.

Klein, G. S. (1976). *Psychoanalytic Theory*. New York, NY: International Universities Press.

Kleinman, A. (1988). *Rethinking Psychiatry: From Cultural Category to Personal Experience*. New York, NY: Free Press.

Klerman, G. L. (1972). Psychotropic hedonism vs. pharmacological Calvinism. *Hastings Center Report*, **2**, 1–3.

Knutson, B., Wolkowitz, O. M. & Cole, S. W. (1998). Selective alteration of personality and social behavior by serotonergic intervention. *American Journal of Psychiatry*, **155**, 373–9.

Kohlberg, L. (1981). *The Philosophy of Moral Development: Moral Stages and the Idea of Justice*. New York, NY: Harper & Row.

Komesaroff, P. A. (1995). *Troubled Bodies: Critical Perspectives on Postmodernism, Medical Ethics, and the Body*. Durham, NC: Duke University Press.

Kopelman, L. M. (1992). Philosophical issues concerning psychiatric diagnosis. *The Journal of Medicine and Philosophy*, **2**, 121–261.

Kovacs, J. (1998). The concept of health and disease. *Medicine, Health Care and Philosophy*, **1**, 31–9.

Kovecses, Z. (1986). *Metaphors of Anger, Pride, and Love: A Lexical Approach to the Structure of Concepts*. Philadelphia, PA: Benjamins.

Kramer, P. D. (1997). *Listening to Prozac*. London: Penguin.

Kriel, J. (2000). *Matter, Mind, and Medicine: Transforming the Clinical Method*. Amsterdam: Rodopi.

Kripke, S. (1980). *Naming and Necessity*. Oxford: Oxford University Press.

Kuhn, T. S. (1971). *The Structure of Scientific Revolutions*, 2nd edn. Chicago, IL: Chicago University Press.

Kurzweil, R. (2005). *The Singularity is Near*. New York, NY: Viking.

Kutchins, H. & Kirk, S. A. (1997). *Making Us Crazy: DSM – The Psychiatric Bible and the Creation of Mental Disorders*. New York, NY: Free Press.

LaFrance, W. C., Lauterbach, E. C., Coffey, E. C., *et al.* (2000). The use of herbal alternative medicines in neuropsychiatry. *Journal of Neuropsychiatry and Clinical Neuroscience*, **12**, 177–92.

Lakatos, I. (1978). *The Methodology of Scientific Research Programmes: Philosophical Papers* (edited by J. Worrall & G. Currie). Cambridge: Cambridge University Press.

Lakoff, A. (2006). *Pharmaceutical Reason: Knowledge and Value in Global Psychiatry.* Cambridge: Cambridge University Press.

Lakoff, G. (1987). *Women, Fire, and Dangerous Things: What Categories Reveal about the Mind.* Chicago, IL: University of Chicago Press.

Lakoff, G. & Johnson, M. (1999). *Philosophy in the Flesh: The Embodied Mind and Its Challenge to Western Thought.* New York, NY: Basic Books.

Laland, K. N. & Brown, G. R. (2002). *Sense and Nonsense: Evolutionary Perspectives on Human Behaviour.* Oxford: Oxford University Press.

Lam, D. C. K., Salkovskis, P. M. & Warwick, H. M. C. (2005). An experimental investigation of the impact of biological versus psychological explanations of the cause of "mental illness". *Journal of Mental Health,* **14**, 453–64.

Landman, W. A. & Henley, L. D. (1998). Tensions in setting health care priorities for South Africa's children. *Journal of Medical Ethics,* **24**, 268–73.

Lane, C. (2007). *Shyness: How Normal Behaviour Became a Sickness.* New Haven, CT: Yale University Press.

Langer, S. (1942). *Philosophy in a New Key.* Cambridge, MA: Havard University Press.

Latour, B. & Woolgar, S. (1992). *Laboratory Life: Construction of Scientific Facts.* Princeton, NJ: Princeton University Press.

Layne, C. (1983). Painful truths about depressive's cognitions. *Journal of Clinical Psychology,* **39**, 848–53.

Le Doux, J. E. (1996). *The Emotional Brain: The Mysterious Underpinnings of Emotional Life.* New York, NY: Simon and Schuster.

Le Doux, J. E. (2002). *Synaptic Self: How Our Brains Become Who We Are.* New York, NY: Viking.

Leary, M. & Tangney, J. P. (2002). *Handbook of Self and Identity.* New York, NY: Guilford Press.

Leary, M. R. (2006). *The Curse of the Self: Self-Awareness, Egotism, and the Quality of Human Life.* Oxford: Oxford University Press.

Leber, P. (2000). The use of placebo control groups in the assessment of psychiatric drugs: an historical context. *Biological Psychiatry,* **47**, 699–706.

Leder, D. (1984). Medicine and paradigms of embodiment. *Journal of Medicine and Philosophy*, **9**, 29–43.

Legrand, D. (2006). The boding self: the sensori-motor roots of pre-reflective self-consciousness. *Phenomenology and the Cognitive Sciences*, **5**, 89–118.

Leuchter, A. F., Cook, I. A., Witte, E. A., Morgan, M. & Abrams, M. (2002). Changes in brain function of depressed patients during treatment with placebo. *American Journal of Psychiatry*, **159**, 122–9.

Levine, J. (1983). Materialism and qualia: the explanatory gap. *Pacific Philosophical Quarterly*, **64**, 354–61.

Levins, R. & Lewontin, R. (1985). *The Dialetical Biologist*. Cambridge, MA: Harvard University Press.

Lewis, B. (2006). *Moving Beyond Prozac, DSM, and the New Psychiatry*. Ann Arbor, MI: University of Michigan Press.

Lewis, D. (1983). *Philosophical Papers*, Vol. 1. Oxford: Oxford University Press.

Libet, B., Freeman, A. & Sutherland, K. (1999). *The Volitional Brain: Towards a Neuroscience of Free Will*. Thorverton, UK: Imprint Academic.

Lightman, A., Sarewitz, D. & Desser, C. (2003). *Living with the Genie: Essays on Technology and the Quest for Human Mastery*. Washington, DC: Island Press.

Lilienfeld, S. O. & Marino, L. (1995). Mental disorder as a Roschian concept: a critique of Wakefield's "harmful dysfunction" analysis. *Journal of Abnormal Psychology*, **104**, 411–20.

Lilienfeld, S. O. & Marino, S. (1999). Essentialism revisited: evolutionary theory and the concept of mental disorder. *Journal of Abnormal Psychology*, **108**, 400–11.

Lippman, A. (1992). Led (astray) by genetic maps: the cartography of the human genome and health care. *Social Science and Medicine*, **35**, 1469–76.

Litton, P. (2005). ADHD, values, and the self. *American Journal of Bioethics*, **5**, 65–7.

Livesley, W. J. (1985). The classification of personality disorder: 1. The choice of category concept. *Canadian Journal of Psychiatry*, **30**, 353–8.

Livesley, W. J. (1986). Trait and behavioral prototypes of personality disorder. *American Journal of Psychiatry*, **143**, 728–32.

Lloyd, D. (2004). *Radiant Cool: A Novel Theory of Consciousness*. Cambridge, MA: Bradford Book/MIT Press.

Lock, M. (1993). *Encounters with Aging: Mythologies of Menopause in Japan and North America*. Berkeley, CA: University of California Press.

Lock, M. & Kaufert, P. A. (1998). *Pragmatic Women and Body Politics*. Cambridge: Cambridge University Press.

Locke, J. (1694). *An Essay Concerning Human Understanding*. Amherst: Prometheus Books [1995].

Longino, H. (1990). *Science as Social Knowledge: Values and Objectivity in Scientific Inquiry*. Princeton, NJ: Princeton University Press.

Lovibond, S. (1983). *Realism and Imagination in Ethics*. Minneapolis, MN: University of Minnesota Press.

Lucas, F. R. (1993). *Responsibility*. Oxford: Clarendon Press.

Luhrmann, T. M. (2000). *Of Two Minds: An Anthropologist Looks at American Psychiatry*. New York, NY: Alfred A. Knopf.

Lyon, W. (1980). *Emotion*. Cambridge: Cambridge University Press.

MacIntyre, A. C. (1981). *After Virtue: A Study in Moral Theory*. Notre Dame, IN: University of Notre Dame Press.

Mackie, J. L. (1976). *Problems from Locke*. Oxford: Oxford University Press.

Macklin, R. (1973). The medical model in psychoanalysis and psychotherapy. *Comprehensive Psychiatry*, **14**, 49–69.

Macklin, R. (1999). *Against Relativism: Cultural Diversity and the Search for Ethical Universals in Medicine*. Oxford: Oxford University Press.

MacLean, P. D. (1985). Evolutionary psychiatry and the triune brain. *Psychological Medicine*, **15**, 219–21.

Malik, K. (2000). *Man, Beast, and Zombie: What Science Can and Cannot Tell Us About Human Nature*. London: Weidefeld and Nicolson.

Manicas, P. T. & Secord, P. F. (1983). Implications for psychology of the new philosophy of science. *American Psychologist*, **38**, 399–413.

Maravita, A., Spence, C. & Driver, J. (2003). Multisensory integration and the body schema: close to hand and within reach. *Current Biology*, **13**, 531–9.

Marcus, S. J. (2002). *Neuroethics: Mapping the Field.* New York, NY: Dana Press.

Mareschal, D., Johnson, M. H., Sirois, S., Spratling, M., Thomas, M. & Westermann, G. (2007). *Neuroconstructivism, Vol. I: How the Brain Constructs Cognition.* Oxford: Oxford University Press.

Margolis, J. (1976). The concept of disease. *Journal of Medicine and Philosophy*, **1**, 238–55.

Margolis, J. (1986). *Pragmatism Without Foundations: Reconciling Realism and Relativism.* Oxford: Basil Blackwell.

Marijuán, P. C. (2001). *Cajal and Consciousness: Scientific Approaches to Consciousness on the Centennial of Ramón y Cajal's Textura.* New York, NY: New York Academy of Sciences.

Marks, J. (2002). *What it Means to be 98% Chimpanzee: Apes, People, and Their Genes.* Berkeley, CA: University of California Press.

Martin, L. H., Gutman, H. & Hutton, P. H. (1988). *Technologies of the Self: A Seminar with Michel Foucault.* Amherst, MA: University of Massachusetts Press.

Martin, R. (1998). *Self-Concern: An Experiential Approach to What Matters in Identity.* Cambridge: Cambridge University Press.

Masters, R. D. & McGuire, M. T. (1994). *The Neurotransmitter Revolution: Serotonin, Social Behavior, and the Law.* Carbondale, SI: Southern Illinois University Press.

Mattay, V. S., Goldberg, T. E., Fera, F., *et al.* (2003). Catechol *O*-methyltransferase val158–met genotype and individual variation in the brain response to amphetamine. *Proceedings of the National Academy of Science USA*, **100**, 6186–91.

Matthews, E. H. (2004). Merleau-Ponty's body-subject and psychiatry. *International Review of Psychiatry*, **16**, 190–8.

May, L., Friedman, M. & Clark, A. (1996). *Mind and Morals: Essays on Ethics and Cognitive Science.* Cambridge, MA: MIT Press.

Mayberg, H. S., Silva, J. A., Brannan, S. K., *et al.* (2002). The functional neuroanatomy of the placebo effect. *American Journal of Psychiatry*, **159**, 728–37.

Mayr, E. (1988). *Towards a New Philosophy of Biology.* Cambridge, MA: Harvard University Press.

McCall Smith, A. (2004). Human action, neuroscience and the law. In D. Rees & S. Rose, eds. *The New Brain Sciences: Perils and Pitfalls.* Cambridge: Cambridge University Press.

McDonald, C. J., Mazzuca, S. A. & McCabe, G. P. J. (1983). How much of the placebo "effect" is really statistical regression? *Statistics in Medicine,* **2**, 417–27.

McDowell, J. (1998). *Mind, Value, and Reality.* Cambridge, MA: Harvard University Press.

McGee, G. (1997). *The Perfect Baby: A Pragmatic Approach to Genetics.* New York, NY: Rowan and Littlefield.

McGinn, C. (1983). *The Subjective View: Secondary Qualities and Indexical Thoughts.* Oxford: Clarendon Press.

McGinn, C. (1989). Can we solve the mind–body problem? *Mind,* **98**, 349–66.

McGinn, C. (1993). *Problems in Philosophy: The Limits of Inquiry.* Oxford: Blackwell Publishing.

McGuire, M. & Troisi, A. (1998). *Darwinian Psychiatry.* New York, NY: Oxford University Press.

McHenry, L. (2006). Ethical issues in psychopharmacology. *Journal of Medical Ethics,* **32**, 405–10.

McHugh, P. R. & Slavney, P. R. (1988). *The Perspectives of Psychiatry.* Baltimore, MA: Johns Hopkins University Press.

McKibben, B. (2003). *Enough: Staying Human in an Engineered Age.* New York, NY: Times.

Mealey, L. (1997). The nature of normality (Reply to Stein). *Behavioral and Brain Sciences,* **20**, 530–1.

Megone, C. (1998). Aristotle's function argument and the concept of mental illness. *Philosophy, Psychiatry & Psychology,* **5**, 187–201.

Megone, C. (2000). Mental illness, human function, and values. *Philosophy, Psychiatry & Psychology,* **7**, 45–65.

Mehlman, M. (2003). *Wonder Genes: Genetic Enhancement and the Future of Society.* Indianapolis, IN: Indianapolis University Press.

Merleau-Ponty, M. (1942). *The Structure of Behaviour.* New York, NY: Beacon Press [1967].

Merleau-Ponty, M. (1962). *Phenomenology of Perception*. London: Routledge and Kegan Paul.

Merleau-Ponty, M. (1963a). *In Praise of Philosophy and Other Essays* (translated by J. Wild, J. Edie & J. O'Neill). Evanston, IL: Northwestern University Press.

Merleau-Ponty, M. (1963b). *The Structure of Behaviour*. New York, NY: Beacon.

Merton, R. K. (1973). *The Sociology of Science: Theoretical and Empirical Investigations*. Chicago, IL: University of Chicago Press.

Metzinger, T. (2003). *Being No One: The Self-Model Theory of Subjectivity*. Cambridge, MA: MIT Press.

Metzl, J. M. (2003). *Prozac on the Couch: Prescribing Gender in the Era of Wonder Drugs*. Durham, NC: Duke University Press.

Metzl, J. M. & Angel, J. (2004). Assessing the impact of SSRI antidepressants on popular notions of women's depressive illness. *Social Science and Medicine*, **58**, 577–84.

Mezzich, J. E. (1989). An empirical prototypical approach to the definition of psychiatric illness. *British Journal of Psychiatry*, **154S4**, 42–6.

Miah, A. (2004). *Genetically Modified Athletes – Biomedical Ethics, Gene Doping and Sport*. London and New York: Routledge.

Midgley, M. (1978). *Beast and Man: The Roots of Human Nature*. London: Routledge.

Mill, J. S. (1843). *A System of Logic*. Honolulu, HI: University Press of the Pacific [2002].

Mill, J. S. (1863). *Utilitarianism*. Indianapolis, IN: Hackett.

Mill, J. S. (1998). *Nature: Three Essays on Religion*. Amherst, MA: Prometheus.

Miller, G. A., Gallanter, E. & Pribram, K. (1960). *Plans and the Structure of Behavior*. New York, NY: Holt, Rinehart and Winston.

Miller, R. B. (1992). *Readings in the Philosophy of Clinical Psychology: The Restoration of Dialogue*. Washington, DC: American Psychological Association.

Miller, R. W. (1987). *Fact and Method: Explanation, Confirmation and Reality in the Natural and the Social Sciences*. Princeton, NJ: Princeton University Press.

Millikan, R. (1984). *Language, Thought and Other Biological Categories: New Foundations for Realism.* Cambridge, MA: MIT Press.

Minsky, M. (2006). *The Emotion Machine: Commonsense Thinking, Artificial Intelligence, and the Future of the Human Mind.* New York, NY: Simon & Schuster.

Mishara, A. (2007). Missing links in phenomenological clinical neuroscience: why we are still not there yet. *Current Opinion in Psychiatry,* **20**, 559–69.

Mitchell, S. A. (1988). *Relational Concepts in Psychoanalysis: An Integration.* Cambridge, MA: Harvard University Press.

Mitchell, S. D. (2003). *Biological Complexity and Integrative Pluralism.* Cambridge: Cambridge University Press.

Moerman, D. E. (2002). *Meaning, Medicine and the 'Placebo Effect'.* Cambridge: Cambridge University Press.

Moore, G. E. (1903). *Principia Ethica.* Cambridge: Cambridge University Press.

Moreno, J. D. (2006a). Juicing the brain. *Scientific American Mind,* **17**, 66–73.

Moreno, J. D. (2006b). *Mind Wars: Brain Science and National Defense.* New York, NY: Dana Press.

Morris, C. (1973). *The Discovery of the Individual 1050–2000.* New York, NY: Harper Torchbooks.

Morris, J. S. (2002). How do you feel? *Trends in Cognitive Sciences,* **6**, 317–19.

Morse, S. J. (2006). Moral and legal responsibility and the new neuroscience. In J. Illes, ed. *Neuroethics: Defining the Issues in Theory, Practice, and Policy.* Oxford: Oxford University Press.

Morton, A. (1980). Character and the emotions. In A. O. Rorty, ed. *Explaining Emotions.* Berkeley and Los Angeles, CA: University of California, pp. 153–62.

Moynihan, R. (2002). Drug firms hype disease as sales ploy, industry chief claims. *British Medical Journal,* **324**, 867.

Moynihan, R. & Henry, D. (2006). The fight against disease mongering: Generating knowledge for action. *PLoS Medicine,* **3**, 191.

Moynihan, R. & Smith, R. (2002). Too much medicine? *British Medical Journal,* **324**, 859–60.

Muller, J. E., Koen, L. & Stein, D. J. (2004). The spectrum of social anxiety disorders. In B. Bandelow & D. J. Stein, eds. *Social Anxiety Disorder.* New York, NY: Marcel Dekker.

Murray, C. J. L. & Lopez, A. D. (1996). *Global Burden of Disease: A Comprehensive Assessment of Mortality and Morbidity from Diseases, Injuries and Risk Factors in 1990 and Projected to 2020,* Vol. I. Harvard, MA: World Health Organization.

Murray, S. J. (2007). Care and the self: biotechnology, reproduction, and the good life. *Philosophy, Ethics and Humanities in Medicine,* 2, 6.

Murray, T. H., Gaylin, W. & Macklin, R. (1984). *Feeling Good and Doing Better: Ethics and Nontherapeutic Drug Use.* Clifton, NJ: Humana Press.

Mwase, I. M. (2005). Genetic enhancement and the fate of the worse off. *Kennedy Institute Ethics Journal,* 15, 83–9.

Naam, R. (2005). *More Than Human: Embracing the Promise of Biological Enhancement.* New York, NY: Broadway Books.

Nagel, T. (1989). *The View from Nowhere.* New York, NY: Oxford University Press.

Narrow, W. E., Rae, D. S., Robins, L. N. & Regier, D. A. (2002). Revised prevalence estimates of mental disorders in the United States. *Archives of General Psychiatry,* 59, 115–23.

Nebert, D. W., Jorge-Nebert, L. & Vesell, E. S. (2003). Pharmacogenomics and "individualized drug therapy": high expectations and disappointing achievements. *American Journal of PharmacoGenomics,* 3, 361–70.

Neisser, U. (1976). *Cognition and Reality.* San Francisco, CA: Freeman.

Neisser, U. (1988). Five kinds of self-knowledge. *The Philosophy of Psychology,* 1, 35–59.

Neisser, U. & Fivush, R. (1994). *The Remembering Self: Construction and Accuracy in the Self-Narrative.* Cambridge: Cambridge University Press.

Nelson, H. L. (1997). *Stories and Their Limits: Narrative Approaches to Bioethics.* New York, NY: Routledge.

Nelson, J. L. (1995). Critical interests and sources of familial decision-making for incapacitated patients. *Journal of Law, Medicine, and Ethics,* 23, 143–8.

Nesse, R. M. (1990). Evolutionary explanations of emotions. *Human Nature,* 1, 261–89.

Nesse, R. M. (2000). Is depression an adaptation? *Archives of General Psychiatry,* **57**, 14–20.

Nesse, R. M. (2001). On the difficulty of defining disease: a Darwinian perspective. *Medicine, Health Care and Philosophy,* **4**, 37–46.

Nesse, R. M. & Berridge, K. C. (1997). Psychoactive drug use in evolutionary perspective. *Science,* **278**, 63–6.

Nesse, R. M. & Williams, G. C. (1994). *Why We Get Sick: The New Science of Darwinian Medicine.* New York, NY: Vintage Books.

Neu, J. (1977). *Emotion, Thought and Therapy: A Study of Hume and Spinoza and the Relationship of Philosophical Theories of the Emotions to Psychological Theories of Therapy.* London: Routledge and Kegan Paul.

Neurath, O., Carnap, R. & Morris, C. (1969). *Foundations of the Unity of Science: Toward an International Encyclopedia of Unified Science.* Chicago, IL: University of Chicago Press.

Nietzche, F. (1968). *The Will to Power* (translated by W. Kaufmann & R. J. Hollingdale). New York, NY: Vintage.

Nightingale, P. & Martin, P. A. (2004). The myth of the biotech revolution. *Trends in Biotechnology,* **22**, 564–9.

Nordenfelt, L. (1995). *On the Nature of Health: An Action-Theoretic Approach.* Boston, MA: Kluwer.

Norman, D. A. (1986). Reflections on cognition and parallel distributed processing cognition. In J. L. McClelland & D. E. Rumelhart, eds. *Parallel Distributed Processing: Explorations in the Microstructure of Cognition,* Vol. 2. Cambridge, MA: MIT Press, pp. 531–52.

Norman, D. A. (1993). Cognition in the head and in the world: an introduction to the special issue on situated action. *Cognitive Science,* **17**, 1–6.

Norman, R. (1996). Interfering with nature. *Journal of Applied Philosophy,* **13**, 1–11.

Northoff, G., Heinzel, A., de Greck, M., Bermpohl, F., Dobrowolny, H. & Panksepp, J. (2006). Self-referential processing in our brain – a meta-analysis of imaging studies on the self. *NeuroImage,* **31**, 440–57.

Nozick, R. (1977). *Anarchy, State, and Utopia.* New York, NY: Basic Books.

Nuffield Council on Bioethics. (2002). *Genetics and Human Behaviour: The Ethical Context.* London: Nuffield Council.

Nussbaum, M. (1990). *Love's Knowledge: Essays on Philosophy and Literature.* Oxford: Oxford University Press.

Nussbaum, M. (2001). *Upheavals of Thought.* New York, NY: Cambridge University Press.

O'Donovan, O. (1984). *Begotten or Made?* Oxford: Clarendon Press.

O'Neill, J. (1985). *Five Bodies: The Human Shape of Modern Society.* Ithaca, NY: Cornell University Press.

O'Regan, J. K. & Noë, A. (2001). A sensorimotor account of vision and visual consciousness. *Behavioral and Brain Sciences,* **24**, 939–1031.

O'Reilly, R. C. (2006). Biologically based computational models of high-level cognition. *Science,* **314**, 91–4.

Oatley, K. & Johnson-Laird, P. (1987). Towards a cognitive theory of emotion. *Cognition and Emotion,* **1**, 29–50.

Olding-Smee, F. J., Laland, K. N. & Feldman, M. W. (2003). *Niche Construction: The Neglected Process in Evolution.* Princeton, NJ: Princeton University Press.

Ott, J. & Hofmann, A. (1996). Pharmacotheon: Entheogenic Drugs, Their Plant Sources and History, 2nd edn. Kennewick, WA: Natural Products Co.

Packard, V. (1977). *The People Shapers.* Boston, MA: Little, Brown & Co.

Pahnke, W. N. (1969). Psychedelic drugs and mystical experience. *International Psychiatric Clinics,* **5**, 149–62.

Panksepp, J. (1998). *Affective Neuroscience: The Foundations of Human and Animal Emotions.* Oxford: Oxford University Press.

Panksepp, J. (2003). Feeling the pain of social loss. *Science,* **302**, 237–9.

Panksepp, J. (2005). Affective consciousness: core emotional feelings in animals and humans. *Consciousness and Cognition,* **14**, 30–80.

Panksepp, J. & Panksepp, J. B. (2000). The seven sins of evolutionary psychology. *Evolution and Cognition,* **6**, 108–31.

Papert, S. (1980). *Mindstorms: Children, Computers, and Powerful Ideas.* Brighton, Sussex: Harvester Press.

Papineau, D. (1993). *Philosophical Naturalism.* Oxford: Blackwell.

Papineau, D. (2003). *The Roots of Reason: Philosophical Essays on Rationality, Evolution, and Probability.* Oxford: Oxford University Press.

Paquetta, V., Lévesquea, J., Mensourb, B., *et al.* (2003). "Change the mind and you change the brain": effects of cognitive-behavioral therapy on the neural correlates of spider phobia. *NeuroImage,* **18**, 401–9.

Parens, E. (1998a). *Enhancing Human Traits: Ethical and Social Implications.* Washington, DC: Georgetown University Press.

Parens, E. (1998b). Is better always good? The enhancement project. In E. Parens, ed. *Enhancing Human Traits.* Washington, DC: Georgetown University Press.

Parens, E. (2004). Genetic differences and human identities: on why talking about behavioral genetics is important and difficult. *Hastings Center Report,* **S34**, 1–35.

Parens, E. (2005). Authenticity and ambivalence: towards understanding the enhancement debate. *Hastings Center Report,* **35**, 34–41.

Parens, E. (2006). *Surgically Shaping Children: Technology, Ethics, and the Pursuit of Normality.* Baltimore, MD: Johns Hopkins University Press.

Parfit, D. (1984). *Reasons and Persons.* Oxford: Clarendon Press.

Parsons, T. (1951). *The Social System.* New York, NY: The Free Press.

Peirce, C. S. (1992). *The Essential Peirce, Selected Philosophical Writings, Vol. 1 (1867–1893)* (edited by N. Houser & C. Kloesel). Bloomington and Indianapolis, IN: Indiana University Press.

Pellegrino, E. (1997). Praxis as a keystone for the philosophy and professional ethics of medicine. In R. Carson & C. Burns, eds. *Philosophy of Medicine and Bioethics.* Dordrecht: Kluwer.

Pellegrino, E. D. (2004). Biotechnology, human enhancement, and the ethics of medicine. *Dignity,* **10**, 1–5.

Pellegrino, E. D. & Thomasma, D. C. (1981). *A Philosophical Basis of Medical Practice.* New York, NY: Oxford University Press.

Pennock, P. E. (2007). *Advertising Sin and Sickness: The Politics of Alcohol and Tobacco Marketing, 1950–1990.* De Kalb, IL: North Illinois University Press.

Perring, C. (1997a). Degrees of personhood. *Journal of Medicine and Philosophy,* **22**, 173–97.

Perring, C. (1997b). Medicating children: the case of Ritalin. *Bioethics,* **11**, 228–40.

Perry, J. (1975). *Personal Identity.* Berkeley and Los Angeles, CA: University of California Press.

Petersen, R. C., Stevens, J. C., Ganguli, M., Tangalos, E. G., Cummings, J. L. & DeKosky, S. T. (2001). Practice parameter: early detection of dementia – mild cognitive impairment (an evidence-based review): report of the Quality Standards Subcommittee of the American Academy of Neurology. *Neurology,* **56**, 1133–42.

Pezawas, L., Meyer-Lindenberg, A., Drabant, E. M., *et al.* (2005). 5-HTTLPR polymorphism impacts human cingulate-amygdala interactions: a genetic susceptibility mechanism for depression. *Nature Neuroscience,* **8**, 828–34.

Phillips, J. (2003). Psychopathology and the narrative self. *Philosophy, Psychiatry & Psychology,* **10**, 313–28.

Phillips, K. A., McElroy, S. L., Keck, P. A., *et al.* (1993). Body dysmorphic disorder: 30 cases of imagined ugliness. *American Journal of Psychiatry,* **150**, 302–8.

Piaget, J. (1952). *The Origins of Intelligence in Children.* New York, NY: International Universities Press.

Piaget, J. (1970). *The Place of the Sciences of Man in the System of Sciences.* New York, NY: Harper & Row.

Piaget, J. (1972a). *Insights and Illusions of Philosophy* (translated by W. Mays). London: Routledge & Kegan Paul.

Piaget, J. (1972b). *Psychology and Epistemology: Towards a Theory of Knowledge.* Harmondsworth, UK: Penguin Books.

Piatelli-Palmarini, M. (1994). *Inevitable Illusions: How Mistakes of Reason Rule our Minds.* New York, NY: John Wiley & Sons.

Piattelli-Palmarini, M. (1980). *Language and Learning: The Debate Between Jean Piaget and Naom Chomsky.* London: Routledge and Kegan Paul.

Picard, R. W. (1997). *Affective Computing.* Cambridge, MA: MIT Press.

Pickering, N. (2006). *The Metaphor of Mental Illness.* Oxford: Oxford University Press.

Pies, R. (2006). Why psychiatry and neurology simply cannot merge. *Journal of Neuropsychiatry and Clinical Neuroscience,* **17**, 304–9.

Pinker, S. (2004). *The Blank Slate: The Modern Denial of Human Nature.* New York, NY: Viking.

Pitman, R. K., Sanders, K. M., Zusman, R. M., *et al.* (2002). Pilot study of secondary prevention of posttraumatic stress disorder with propranolol. *Biological Psychiatry,* **51**, 189–92.

Plato. (1970). *The Laws*. New York, NY: Penguin Books.

Plato. (1997). *Alcibiades*. In J. M. Cooper, ed. *Complete Works*. Indianapolis and Cambridge: Hackett Publishing.

Plato. (2003). *Phaedrus* (translated by R. Waterfield). New York, NY: Oxford University Press.

Playfair, G. L. (1987). *Medicine, Mind & Magic*. New York, NY: HarperCollins.

Polanyi, M. (1958). *Personal Knowledge: Towards a Post-Critical Philosophy*. London: Routledge and Kegan Paul.

Popper, K. (1974). *Unended Quest*. London: Fontana.

Porter, R. (1997). *The Greatest Benefit to Mankind*. New York, NY: WW Norton.

Post, S. G. & Binstock, R. H. (2004). *The Fountain of Youth: Cultural, Scientific, and Ethical Perspectives on a Biomedical Goal*. New York, NY: Oxford University Press.

Potter, V. R. (1971). *Bioethics: Bridge to the Future*. Englewood Cliffs, NJ: Prentice-Hall.

Power, M. & Dalgleish, T. (1997). *Cognition and Emotion: From Order to Disorder*. Hove: Erlbaum.

President's Council on Bioethics. (2003). *Beyond Therapy: Biotechnology and the Pursuit of Happiness*. Washington, DC: Dana Press.

Prinz, J. (2004). *Gut Reactions: A Perceptual Theory of Emotion*. Oxford: Oxford University Press.

Putnam, H. (1967). The nature of mental states. In W. H. Capitan and D. D. Merill, eds. *Art, Mind, and Religion*. Pittsburgh, PA: University of Pittsburgh Press.

Putnam, H. (1975). *Mind, Language and Reality*. Cambridge: Cambridge University Press.

Putnam, H. (1984). What is realism? In J. Leplin, ed. *Scientific Realism*. Berkeley and Los Angeles, CA: University of California Press.

Putnam, H. (2002). *The Collapse of the Fact/Value Dichotomy and Other Essays*. Cambridge, MA: Harvard University Press.

Quine, W. V. O. (1960). *Word and Object*. Cambridge, MA: MIT Press.

Quine, W. V. O. (1969). *Epistemology Naturalized. Ontological Relativity and Other Essays*. New York, NY: Columbia University Press.

Quinton, A. (1962). The Soul. *The Journal of Philosophy*, **59**, 393–409.

Radden, J. (1996). *Divided Minds and Successive Selves: Ethical Issues in Disorders of Identity and Personality*. Cambridge, MA: MIT Press.

Radden, J. (2000). *The Nature of Melancholy: From Aristotle to Kristeva*. Oxford: Oxford University Press.

Radden, J. H. (2004). *The Philosophy of Psychiatry: A Companion*. Oxford: Oxford University Press.

Ramsay, W., Stitch, S. & Rumelhart, D. (1991). *Philosophy and Connectionist Theory*. Hillsdale, NJ: Lawrence Erlbaum.

Rapoport, J. L., Ryland, D. H. & Kriete, M. (1992). Drug treatment of canine acral lick. *Archives of General Psychiatry*, **48**, 517–21.

Rapp, R. (2000). *Testing Women, Testing the Fetus: The Social Impact of Amniocentesis in America*. New York, NY: Routledge.

Rauch, S. L., Shin, L. M., Whalen, P. J. & Pitman, R. K. (1998). Neuroimaging and the neuroanatomy of posttraumatic stress disorder. *CNS Spectrums*, **3**, 31–41.

Rawls, J. (1971). *A Theory of Justice*. Cambridge, MA: Harvard University Press.

Raymond, J. G. (1993). *Women as Wombs: Reproductive Technologies and the Battle over Women's Freedom*. New York, NY: Harper Collins.

Rees, D. & Rose, S. (2004). *The New Brain Sciences: Perils and Prospects*. Cambridge: Cambridge University Press.

Rego, M. D. (2005). What are (and what are not) the existential implications of antidepressant use? *Philosophy, Psychiatry and Psychology*, **12**, 119–28.

Reiser, S. J. (1978). *Medicine and the Reign of Technology*. New York, NY: Cambridge University Press.

Reiss, M. J. & Straughan, R. (1996). *Improving Nature?The Science and Ethics of Genetic Engineering*. Cambridge: Cambridge University Press.

Resnik, D., Steinkraus, H. & Langer, P. (1999). *Human Germline Gene Therapy*. Austin, TX: Landes Bioscience.

Resnik, D. B. & Vorhaus, D. B. (2006). Genetic modification and genetic determinism. *Philosophy, Ethics and Humanities in Medicine*, **1**, 9.

Restak, R. (2003). *The New Brain: How the Modern Age is Rewiring Your Mind*. New York, NY: Rodale Books.

Rey, G. (1980). Functionalism and the emotions. In A. O. Rorty, ed. *Explaining Emotions*. Berkeley and Los Angeles, CA: University of California Press, pp. 163–95.

Reynolds, V. (1976). *The Biology of Human Action.* Oxford: W. H. Freeman and Company.

Reznek, L. (1988). *Nature of Disease.* London: Routledge.

Reznek, L. (1991). *The Philosophical Defence of Psychiatry.* London: Routledge.

Reznek, L. (1997). *Evil or Ill? Justifying the Insanity Defence.* London: Routledge.

Richards, J. R. (2000). *Human Nature After Darwin: A Philosophical Introduction.* London: Routledge.

Ricoeur, P. (1970). *Freud and Philosophy: An Essay on Interpretation.* New Haven, CT: Yale University Press.

Ricoeur, P. (1981). *Hermeneutics and the Human Sciences: Essays on Language, Action and Interpretation.* Cambridge: Cambridge University Press.

Ricoeur, P. (1992). *Onself as Another.* Chicago, IL: University of Chicago Press.

Ridley, M. (2003). *Nature via Nurture.* London: Harper Collins.

Rieff, P. (1979). *Freud: The Mind of the Moralist,* 3rd edn. Chicago, IL: University of Chicago Press.

Rifken, J. (1983). *Algeny.* New York, NY: Viking Books.

Rifkin, J. (1998). *The Biotech Century: Harnessing the Gene and Remaking the World.* London: Gollancz.

Rivers, W. H. R. (2001). *Medicine, Magic and Religion.* London: Routledge.

Roberts, R. (2003). *Emotions: An Essay in Aid of Moral Psychology.* Cambridge: Cambridge University Press.

Robertson, J. (1994). *Children of Choice.* Princeton, NJ: Princeton University Press.

Rochat, P. (1995). *The Self in Infancy: Theory and Research.* Amsterdam: Elsevier.

Rodriguez, A., Aregullin, M., Nishida, T., *et al.* (1985). Thiarubrine A, a bioactive constituent of *Aspilia* (Asteraceae) consumed by wild chimpanzees. *Experientia,* **15**, 419–20.

Roffman, J. L., Marci, D., Glick, D. M., Dougherty, D. D. & Rauch, S. L. (2005). Neuroimaging and the functional neuroanatomy of psychotherapy. *Psychological Medicine,* **35**, 1385–98.

Rorty, A. (1975). *The Identities of Persons.* Berkeley, CA: University of California Press.

Rorty, A. O. (1980). *Explaining Emotions.* Berkeley and Los Angeles, CA: University of California Press.

Rorty, R. (1979). *Philosophy and the Mirror of Nature.* Princeton, NJ: Princeton University Press.

Rosch, E. (1978). Principles of categorization. In E. Rosch & B. B. Lloyd, eds. *Cognition and Categorization.* Hillsdale, NJ: Lawrence Erlbaum Associates.

Rose, H. & Rose, S. (2000). *Alas Poor Darwin: Arguments Against Evolutionary Psychology.* New York, NY: Random House.

Rose, N. (1998a). *Inventing Our Selves: Psychology, Power, and Personhood.* Cambridge: Cambridge University Press.

Rose, N. (2007). *The Politics of Life Itself: Biomedicine, Power, and Subjectivity in the Twenty-First Century.* Princeton, NJ: Princeton University Press.

Rose, S. (1998b). *Lifelines: Biology Beyond Determinism.* Oxford: Oxford University Press.

Rose, S., Bisson, J., Churchill, R. & Wessely, S. (2002). Psychological debriefing for preventing post traumatic stress disorder (PTSD). *Cochrane Database System Reviews,* CD000560.

Rose, S. & The Dialectics of Biology Group. (1982). *Towards a Liberation Biology.* New York, NY: Allison & Busby.

Rose, S. P. R. (2002). "Smart drugs": do they work? Are they ethical? Will they be legal? *Nature Reviews Neuroscience,* **3**, 975–9.

Rosen, R. D. (1977). *Psychobabble.* New York, NY: Atheneum.

Roth, M. & Kroll, J. (1986). *The Reality of Mental Illness.* Cambridge: Cambridge University Press.

Rothman, D. J. (1991). *Strangers at the Bedside.* New York, NY: Basic Books.

Rothman, D. J. (1997). *Beginnings Count: The Technological Imperative in American Health.* New York, NY: Oxford University Press.

Rothman, S. M. & Rothman, D. J. (2003). *The Pursuit of Perfection: The Promise and Perils of Medical Enhancement.* New York, NY: Pantheon Books.

Rothstein, M. A. (2003). *Pharmacogenomics: Social, Ethical, and Clinical Dimensions.* Hoboken, NJ: Wiley-Liss.

Rounsaville, B. J., Alarcón, R. D., Andrews, G., Jackson, J. S., Kendell, R. E. & Kendler, K. (2002). Basic nomenclature issues for DSM-V. In D. Kupfer, M. B. First & D. E. Regier, eds. *A Research Agenda for DSM-V*. Washington, DC: American Psychiatric Association.

Roy, D. (2005). Grounding words in perception and action: computation insights. *Trends in Cognitive Sciences,* **9**, 389–96.

Rumelhart, D. E., Smolensky, P., McClelland, J. L. & Hinton, G. E. (1986). Schemata and sequential thought processes in PDP models. In J. L. McClelland & D. E. Rumelhart, eds. *Parallel Distributed Processing: Explorations in the Microstructure of Cognition*, Vol. 2. Cambridge, MA: MIT Press, pp. 7–57.

Ruse, M. (1971). Functional statements in biology. *Philosophy of Science,* **38**, 87–95.

Ruse, M. (1979). *Sociobiology: Sense or Nonsense?* Hingham, MA: Kluwer Boston.

Ruse, M. (1989). *Philosophy of Biology Today*. Albany, NY: State University of New York Press.

Ruse, M. (1995). *Evolutionary Naturalism*. London: Routledge.

Ruse, M. (2003). *Darwin and Design: Does Evolution Have a Purpose?* Cambridge, MA: Harvard University Press.

Russell, B. (1912). *The Problems of Philosophy*. New York, NY: Oxford University Press.

Russell, J. (1991). In defense of a prototype approach to emotion concepts. *Journal of Personality and Social Psychology,* **60**, 37–47.

Russell, K., Wilson, M. & Hall, R. (1992). *The Color Complex: The Politics of Skin Color among African Americans*. New York, NY: Doubleday.

Ryle, G. (1949). *The Concept of Mind*. Chicago, IL: University of Chicago Press.

Sabin, J. E. & Daniels, N. (1994). Determining "medical necessity" in mental health practice. *Hastings Center Report,* **24**, 5–13.

Sabshin, M. (1990). Turning points in twentieth-century American psychiatry. *American Journal of Psychiatry,* **147**, 1267–74.

Sackett, D. L., Rosenberg, W. M. C., Muir Gray, J. A. & Richards, W. S. (1996). Evidence-based medicine: what it is and what it isn't. *British Medical Journal,* **312**, 71–2.

Sadegh-Zadeh, K. (2005). Fuzzy health, illness, and disease. *Journal of Medicine and Philosophy,* **25**, 605–38.

Sadler, J. (2005). *Values and Psychiatric Diagnosis.* Oxford: Oxford University Press.

Sadler, J. Z. (1997). Recognizing values: a descriptive–causal method for medical/scientific discourses. *Journal of Medicine and Philosophy,* **22**, 541–65.

Sadler, J. Z. (2002). *Descriptions and Prescriptions: Values, Mental Disorders, and the DSMs.* Baltimore, MD: Johns Hopkins University Press.

Sadler, J. Z. (2003). Mental health II: issues in diagnosis. In S. F. Post, ed. *The Encyclopedia of Bioethics,* 3rd edn. New York, NY: MacMillan Reference USA, pp. 1810–15.

Sadler, J. Z. & Agich, G. (1995). Diseases, functions, values and psychiatric classification. *Philosophy, Psychiatry & Psychology,* **2**, 219–31.

Sadler, J. Z., Wiggins, O. P. & Schwartz, M. A. (1994). *Philosophical Perspectives on Psychiatric Diagnostic Classification.* Baltimore, MD: Johns Hopkins University Press.

Sala, S. D. (1999). *Mind Myths: Exploring Popular Assumptions about the Mind and Brain.* Chichester, West Sussex: John Wiley & Sons.

Sandel, M. J. (2004). The case against perfection: what's wrong with designer children, bionic athletes, and genetic engineering. *The Atlantic Monthly,* **293**, 51–62.

Sandel, M. J. (2007). *The Case Against Perfection: Ethics in the Age of Genetic Engineering.* Cambridge, MA: Harvard University Press.

Sarkar, S. (2005). *Molecular Models of Life: Philosophical Papers on Molecular Biology.* Cambridge, MA: MIT Press.

Sartre, J.-P. (1948). *The Emotions: Outline of a Theory.* New York, NY: Philosophical Library.

Sayer, A. (2000). *Realism and Social Science.* London: Sage.

Sayre-McCord, G. (2005). Moral realism. In *The Stanford Encyclopedia of Philosophy,* edited by E. N. Zalta. Stanford, CA: The Metaphysics Research Lab. http://plato.stanford.ed

Scadding, J. G. (1967). Diagnosis: the clinician and the computer. *Lancet,* **2**, 877–82.

Schafer, R. (1976). *A New Language for Psychoanalysis.* New Haven, CT: Yale University Press.

Schaffner, K. F. (1994). Psychiatry and molecular biology: Reductionistic approaches to schizophrenia. In J. Z. Sadler, O. P. Wiggins and M. A. Schwartz, eds. *Philosophical Perspectives on Psychiatric Diagnostic Classification.* Baltimore, MD, The Johns Hopkins University Press.

Schaffner, K. F. (1999). Coming home to Hume: a sociobiological foundation for a concept of "health" and morality. *Journal of Medicine and Philosophy,* **24**, 365–75.

Schaler, J. A. (2004). *Szasz Under Fire: The Psychiatric Abolitionist Faces His Critics.* Chicago, IL: Open Court Publishers.

Schechtman, M. (1996). *The Constitution of Selves.* Ithaca, NY: Cornell University Press.

Schermer, M. H. N. (2007). *Brave New World* versus *Island* – utopian and dystopian views on psychopharmacology. *Medicine, Health Care, and Philosophy,* **10**, 119–28.

Schneier, F. R., Blanco, C., Antia, S. X., & Liebowitz, M. R. (2002). The social anxiety spectrum. *Psychiatric Clinics North America,* **25**, 757–74.

Schopenhauer, A. (1965). *On the Basis of Morality* (translated by A. F. J. Payne). Indianapolis, IN: Bobbs-Merrill.

Schore, A. N. (1994). *Affect Regulation and the Origin of the Self: The Neurobiology of Emotional Development.* Hillside, NJ: Lawrence Erlbaum.

Schulkin, J. (2004). *Bodily Sensibility: Intelligent Action.* Oxford: Oxford University Press.

Schramme, T. & Thome, J. (2004). *Philosophy and Psychiatry.* Berlin: De Gruyter.

Schwartz, C. E., Wright, C. I., Shin, L. M., Kagan, J. & Rauch, S. L. (2003). Inhibited and uninhibited infants "grown up": adult amygdalar response to novelty. *Science,* **5627**, 1952–53.

Schwartz, M. A. & Wiggins, O. P. (1986). Systems and the structuring of meaning: contributions to a biopsychosocial medicine. *American Journal of Psychiatry,* **143**, 1213–21.

Schwartz, M. A. & Wiggins, O. P. (1987). Diagnosis and ideal types: a contribution to psychiatric classification. *Comprehensive Psychiatry,* **28**, 277–91.

Schwartz, R. A. (1991). Mood brighteners, affect tolerance, and the blues. *Psychiatry,* **54**, 397–403.

Seaman, B. (2003). *The Greatest Experiment Ever Performed on Women: Exploding the Estrogen Myth.* New York, NY: Hyperion.

Searle, J. (1983). *Intentionality: An Essay in the Philosophy of Mind.* Cambridge: Cambridge University Press.

Searle, J. R. (2006). *Freedom and Neurobiology: Reflections on Free Will, Language, and Political Power.* New York, NY: Columbia University Press.

Sedgwick, P. (1982). *Psychopolitics.* London: Pluto Press.

Seedat, S., Stein, D. J., Berk, M. & Wilson, Z. (2002). Barriers to treatment among members of a mental health advocacy group in South Africa. *Social Psychiatry and Psychiatric Epidemiology*, **37**, 483–7.

Seigel, J. (2005). *The Idea of the Self: Thought and Experience in Western Europe since the Seventeenth Century.* Cambridge: Cambridge University Press.

Selby, M. (2003). Psychiatric resident conceptualizations of mood and affect within the mental status examination. *American Journal of Psychiatry*, **160**, 1527–9.

Sellars, W. (1963). *Science, Perception, and Reality.* New York, NY: Routledge and Kegan Paul.

Shapiro, A. K. & Shapiro, E. (2001). *The Powerful Placebo: From Ancient Priest to Modern Physician.* Baltimore, MD: Johns Hopkins University Press.

Shildrick, M. & Mykitiuk, R. (2005). *Ethics of the Body: Postconventional Challenges.* Cambridge, MA: MIT Press.

Shorter, E. (1998). *A History of Psychiatry: From the Era of the Asylum to the Age of Prozac.* New York, NY: Wiley.

Shotter, J. (1975). *Images of Man in Psychological Research.* London: Methuen.

Showalter, E. (1987). *The Female Malady: Women, Madness, and English Culture, 1830–1980.* New York, NY: Penguin.

Shrader-Frechette, K. & Westra, L. (1997). *Technology and Values.* Lanham, MD: Rowman & Littlefield Publishers.

Shweder, R. & Bourne, E. (1991). Does the concept of the person vary cross-culturally? In R. Shweder, ed. *Thinking Through Cultures: Expeditions in Cultural Psychology.* Cambridge, MA: Harvard University Press.

Siever, L. J. & Davis, K. L. (1991). A psychobiological perspective on the personality disorders. *American Journal of Psychiatry,* **148**, 1647–58.

Silver, L. M. (1998). *Remaking Eden: How Genetic Engineering and Cloning Will Transform the American Family.* New York, NY: Avalon Books.

Simon, B. (1978). *Mind and Madness in Ancient Greece: The Classical Roots of Modern Psychiatry.* Ithaca and London: Cornell University Press.

Singer, P. (1993). *Practical Ethics,* 2nd edn. Cambridge: Cambridge University Press.

Singh, I. (2005). Will the "real boy" please behave: dosing dilemmas for parents of boys with ADHD. *American Journal of Bioethics,* **5**, 34–47.

Slavney, P. R. (1991). Affective disorders: the new imperium. *Comprehensive Psychiatry,* **32**, 295–301.

Small, D. (1984). *Illusion and Reality: The Meaning of Anxiety.* London: J. M. Dent & Sons.

Smith, A. (2002). *A Theory of Moral Sentiment.* New York, NY: Cambridge University Press.

Smith, E. E. & Medin, D. L. (1981). *Categories and Concepts.* Cambridge, MA: Harvard University Press.

Smith, M. (1991). *A Social History of the Minor Tranquilizers.* Binghampton, NY: Pharmaceutical Products Press.

Snodgrass, J. G. & Thompson, R. L. (1997). *The Self Across Psychology: Self-Recognition, Self-Awareness, and the Self Concept.* New York, NY: New York Academy of Sciences.

Solms, M. & Turnbull, O. (2003). *The Brain and the Inner World: An Introduction to the Neuroscience of Subjective Experience.* New York, NY: Other Press.

Solomon, R. (1993). *The Passions: Emotions and the Meaning of Life.* Indianapolis, IN: Hackett.

Solomon, R. (2004). *Thinking about Feeling: Contemporary Philosophers on Emotion.* Oxford: Oxford University Press.

Sommers, C. H. & Satel, S. (2004). *One Nation Under Therapy.* New York, NY: St. Martin's Press.

Sontag, S. (1977). *Illness as Metaphor.* Harmondsworth, England: Penguin.

Spence, S. A., Hunter, M. D. & Harpin, G. (2002). Neuroscience and the will. *Current Opinion in Psychiatry,* **15**, 519–26.

Spitzer, R. L. & Endicott, J. (1978). Medical and mental disorder: proposed definition and criteria. In R. L. Spitzer & D. F. Klein, eds. *Critical Issues in Psychiatric Diagnosis*. New York, NY: Raven Press, pp. 15–39.

Spitzer, R. L. & Wakefield, J. C. (1999). DSM-IV diagnostic criterion for clinical significance: does it help solve the false positive problem? *American Journal of Psychiatry*, **156**, 1856–64.

Staiano, K. (1979). A semiotic definition of illness. *Semiotica*, **28**, 107–25.

Starcevic, V. (2002). Opportunistic "rediscovery" of mental disorders by pharmaceutical industry. *Psychotherapy and Psychosomatics*, **71**, 305–10.

Stein, D. J. (1991). Philosophy and the DSM-III. *Comprehensive Psychiatry*, **32**, 404–15.

Stein, D. J. (1992). Psychoanalysis and cognitive science: contrasting models of the mind. *Journal of the American Academy of Psychoanalysis*, **20**, 543–59.

Stein, D. J. (1993). Cross-cultural psychiatry and the DSM-IV. *Comprehensive Psychiatry*, **34**, 322–9.

Stein, D. J. (1996a). Philosophy of psychopathy. *Perspectives in Biology and Medicine*, **39**, 569–80.

Stein, D. J. (1997). *Cognitive Science and the Unconscious*. Washington, DC: American Psychiatric Press.

Stein, D. J. (1998). Steps towards a comparative clinical psychopharmacology. In N. H. Dodman & L. Shuster, eds. *Textbook of Veterinary Psychopharmacology*. London: Blackwell Press.

Stein, D. J. (2001). Neurobiology of the obsessive–compulsive spectrum of disorders. *Biological Psychiatry*, **47**, 296–304.

Stein, D. J. (2002). Seminar on obsessive–compulsive disorder. *Lancet*, **360**, 397–405.

Stein, D. J. (2003). *Cognitive-Affective Neuroscience of Mood and Anxiety Disorders*. London: Martin Dunitz.

Stein, D. J. (2005). Empathy: at the heart of the mind. *CNS Spectrums*, **10**, 280–3.

Stein, D. J. (2006). Evolutionary theory, psychiatry, and psychopharmacology. *Progress In Neuro-Psychopharmacology & Biological Psychiatry*, **30**, 766–73.

Stein, D. J. & Bouwer, C. (1997). A neuro-evolutionary approach to the anxiety disorders. *Journal of Anxiety Disorders*, **11**, 409–29.

Stein, D. J., Lerer, B. & Stahl, S. (2005). *Evidence-Based Psychopharmacology*. Cambridge: Cambridge University Press.

Stein, D. J. & Matsunaga, H. (2001). Cross-cultural aspects of social anxiety disorder. *Psychiatric Clinics of North America*, **24**, 773–82.

Stein, D. J. & Mayberg, H. (2005). Placebo: the best pill of all. *CNS Spectrums*, **10**, 440–2.

Stein, D. J., Newman, T. K., Savitz, J. & Ramesar, R. (2006). Warriors vs worriers: the role of COMT gene variants. *CNS Spectrums*, **11**, 745–8.

Stein, D. J., Schatzberg, A. & Kupfer, D. (2006). *Textbook of Mood Disorders*. Washington, DC: American Psychiatric Publishing.

Stein, D. J., Seedat, S., Iversen, A. & Wessely, S. (2007). Post-traumatic stress disorder: medicine and politics. *Lancet*, **369**, 139–44.

Stein, D. J., Solms, M. & van Honk, J. (2006). The cognitive-affective neuroscience of the unconscious. *CNS Spectrums*, **11**, 580–3.

Stein, D. J. (1994). Is impulsive aggression a disorder of the individual or a social ill? A matter of metaphor. *Biological Psychiatry*, **36**, 353–5.

Stein, D. J. & Gureje, O. (2004). Depression and anxiety in the developing world: is it time to medicalise the suffering? *Lancet*, **364**, 233–4.

Stein, M. B. (1996b). How shy is too shy? *Lancet*, **347**, 1131–2.

Stein, M. B., Walker, J. R. & Forde, D. R. (1994). Setting diagnostic thresholds for social phobia: considerations from a community survey. *American Journal of Psychiatry*, **151**, 408–12.

Stempsey, W. E. (2004). The philosophy of medicine: development of a discipline. *Medicine, Health Care and Philosophy*, **7**, 243–51.

Stephens, G. L. & Graham, G. (2000). *When Self-Consciousness Breaks: Alien Voices and Inserted Thoughts*. Cambridge, MA: MIT Press.

Stern, D. A. (2000). *The Interpersonal World of the Infant: A View from Psychoanalysis and Developmental Psychology*. New York, NY: Basic Books.

Stevens, A. & Price, J. (1996). *Evolutionary Psychiatry: A New Beginning*. London: Routledge.

Stevens, M. L. (2000). *Bioethics in America: Origins and Cultural Politics*. Baltimore, MD: Johns Hopkins Press.

Stich, S. (1993). Moral philosophy and mental representation. In M. Hechter, L. Nadel & R. E. Michod, eds. *The Origin of Values*. New York, NY: Aldine de Gruyter.

Stivers, R. (2004). *Shades of Loneliness: Pathologies of a Technological Society*. Lanham, MD: Rowman & Littlefield.

Stock, G. (2002). *Redesigning Humans: Our Inevitable Genetic Future*. Boston, MA: Houghton Mifflin.

Stock, G. & Campbell, J. (2000). *Engineering the Human Germline: An Exploration of the Science and Ethics of Altering the Genes We Pass to Our Children*. New York, NY: Oxford University Press.

Stoker, M. & Hegeman, E. (1992). *Valuing Emotions*. Cambridge: Cambridge University Press.

Strasser, S. (1985). *Understanding and Explanation: Basic Ideas Concerning the Humanity of the Human Sciences*. Pittsburgh, PA: Duquesne University Press.

Straube, T., Glauer, M., Dilger, S., Mentzel, H. J. & Miltner, W. H. (2006). Effects of cognitive-behavioral therapy on brain activation in specific phobia. *NeuroImage*, **29**, 123–35.

Straus, E. (1963). *The Primary World of Senses*. Glencoe, NY: The Free Press of Glencoe.

Strawson, G. (1997). The self. *Journal of Consciousness Studies*, **4**, 405–428.

Strawson, P. (1974). *Freedom and Resentment and Other Essays*. London: Metheun.

Strawson, P. (1977). *Individuals: An Essay in Descriptive Metaphysics*. Oxford: Oxford University Press.

Strawson, P. F. (1985). *Skepticism and Naturalism: Some Varieties*. New York, NY: Colombia University Press.

Suppe, F. (1974). The search for philosophic understanding of scientific theories. In F. Suppe, ed. *The Structure of Scientific Theories*. Urbana, IL: University of Illinois Press.

Svenaeus, F. (2007). Do antidepressants affect the self? A phenomenological approach. *Medicine, Health Care, and Philosophy*, **10**, 153–66.

Svensson, T. (1990). *On the Notion of Mental Illness: Problematizing the Medical-Model Conception of Certain Abnormal Behaviour and Mental Afflictions*. Linköping: Sweden: Department of Health and Society.

Szasz, T. (1972). *The Myth of Mental Illness*. London: Paladin.

Szasz, T. (2001). *Pharmacracy: Medicine and Politics in America.* Westpart, CT: Praeger.

Tam, H. (1996). *Punishment, Excuses and Moral Development.* Aldershot: Avebury Press.

Tamburrini, C. (2006). Are doping sanctions justified? A moral relativistic view. *Sport in Society,* **9**, 199–211.

Tancredi, L. R. (2005). *Hardwired Behavior: What Neuroscience Reveals about Morality.* Cambridge: Cambridge University Press.

Tani, J. (1998). An interpretation of the "self" from the dynamical systems perspective: a constructivist approach. *Journal of Consciousness Studies,* **5**, 516–42.

Tånnsjö, T. & Tamburrini, C. (2000). *Values in Sport – Elitism, Nationalism, Gender Equality and the Scientific Manufacture of Winners.* London and New York: E & FN Spon.

Tauber, A. I. (2006). *Patient Autonomy and the Ethics of Responsibility.* Cambridge, MA: MIT Press.

Taylor, C. (1989). *Sources of the Self: The Making of the Modern Identity.* Cambridge, MA: Harvard University Press.

Taylor, D. (2006). *Ginseng, the Divine Root: The Curious History of the Plant that Captivated the World.* Chapel Hill, NC: Algonquin Books.

Tedeschi, R. G., Park, C. L. & Calhoun, L. G. (1998). *Posttraumatic Growth: Positive Changes in the Aftermath of Crisis.* Mahwah, NJ: Lawrence Erlbaum Associates.

Tengland, P.-A. (2001). *Mental Health: A Philosophical Analysis.* Dordrecht: Kluwer Academic Publishers.

Thagard, P. (1993). *Computational Philosophy of Science.* Cambridge, MA: MIT Press.

Thagard, P. (2000). *How Scientists Explain Disease.* Princeton, NJ: Princeton University Press.

Thagard, P. (2006). *Hot Thought: Mechanisms and Applications of Emotional Cognition.* Cambridge, MA: MIT Press.

Thalberg, I. (1997). *Perception, Emotion, and Action.* New Haven, CT: Yale University Press.

Thompson, J. B. (1984). *Studies in the Theory of Ideology.* Cambridge: Polity Press.

Thornton, T. (2000). Mental illness and reductionism: can functions be naturalized? *Philosophy, Psychiatry & Psychology, 7*, 77–94.

Thornton, T. (2002). Reliability and validity in psychiatric classification: values and neo-Humeanism. *Philosophy, Psychiatry & Psychology, 9*, 229–35.

Thornton, T. (2003). Psychopathology and two kinds of narrative account of the self. *Philosophy, Psychiatry & Psychology, 10*, 361–7.

Thornton, T. (2007a). *Essential Philosophy of Psychiatry*. Oxford: Oxford University Press.

Thornton, T. (2007b). The unexamined life is not worth living: philosophy as a natural component of self-conscious psychiatric practice. *Bulletin of the Association for the Advancement of Philosophy and Psychiatry, 14*, 10–13.

Thullier, J. (1999). *Ten Years Which Changed the Face of Mental Illness*. London: Informa Healthcare.

Toulmin, S. (1982). How medicine saved the life of ethics. *Perspectives in Biology and Medicine, 25*, 736–50.

Toulmin, S. (1997). *The Primacy of Practice: Medicine and Post-Modernism* (edited by R. Carson & C. Burns). Dordrecht: Kluwer.

Toulmin, S. (2001). *Return to Reason*. Cambridge, MA: Harvard University Press.

Troisi, A. (2005). The concept of alternative strategies and its relevance to psychiatry and clinical psychology. *Neuroscience and Biobehavioral Reviews, 29*, 159–68.

Tse, W. S. & Bond, A. J. (2002). Serotonergic intervention affects both social dominance and affiliative behaviour. *Psychopharmacology, 161*, 324–30.

Turkle, S. (2004). Whither psychoanalysis in computer software. *Psychoanalytic Psychology, 21*, 16–30.

Turner, L. (2004). Biotechnology, bioethics and anti-aging interventions. *Trends in Biotechnology, 22*, 219–21.

Tyrer, P. & Steinberg, D. (2005). *Models for Mental Disorder: Conceptual Models in Psychiatry*, 3rd edn. Chichester: John Wiley & Sons.

Valenstein, E. S. (1998). *Blaming the Brain: The Truth about Drugs and Mental Health*. New York, NY: Free Press.

Valentine, E. R. (1982). *Conceptual Issues in Psychology*. London: George Allen & Unwin.

van Delden, J., Bolt, I., Kalis, A., Derijks, J. & Leufkens, H. (2004). Tailor-made pharmacotherapy: future developments and ethical challenges in the field of pharmacogenomics. *Bioethics,* **18**, 303–21.

van Leeuwen, E. & Kimsma, G. K. (1997). Philosophy of medical practice: a discursive approach. *Theoretical Medicine,* **18**, 99–112.

van Niekerk, A. A. (1986). The nature and knowledge of persons. *South African Journal of Philosophy,* 5, 9–14.

van Niekerk, A. A. (1989). Beyond the *erklären–verstehen* dichotomy. *South African Journal of Philosophy,* 8, 198–213.

van Praag, H. M. (1998). Inflationary tendencies in judging the yield of depression research. *Neuropsychobiology,* **37**, 130–41.

van Praag, H. M. (2000). Nosologomania: a disorder of psychiatry. *World Journal of Biological Psychiatry,* **1**, 151–8.

van Praag, H. M. (2001). Past expectations, present disappointments, future hopes or psychopathology as the rate-limiting step of progress in psychopharmacology. *Human Psychopharmacology,* **16**, 3–7.

van Staden, C. W. (2006). Mind, brain and person: reviewing psychiatry's constituency. *South African Psychiatry Review,* **9**, 93–6.

Varela, F. J., Thompson, E. & Rosch, E. (1991). *The Embodied Mind: Cognitive Science and Human Experience*. Cambridge, MA: MIT Press.

Vastag, B. (2004). Poised to challenge need for sleep, "wakefulness enhancer" rouses concerns. *Journal of the American Medical Association,* **291**, 167–70.

Velleman, J. D. (2006). *Self to Self: Selected Essays*. Cambridge: Cambridge University Press.

von Wright, G. H. (1971). *Explanation and Understanding*. Ithaca, NY: Cornell University Press.

Vygotsky, L. (1934). *Thinking and Speaking* (translated and edited by E. Hanfmann & G. Vakar), 1962. Cambridge, MA: MIT Press.

Wailoo, K. & Pemberton, S. (2006). *The Troubled Dream of Genetic Medicine: Ethnicity and Innovation in Tay-Sachs, Cystic Fibrosis, and Sickle Cell Disease*. Baltimore, MD: Johns Hopkins University Press.

Wakefield, J. C. (1992a). Disorder as harmful dysfunction: a conceptual critique of DSM-III-R's definition of mental disorder. *Psychology Reviews, 99,* 232–47.

Wakefield, J. C. (1992b). The concept of mental disorder: on the boundary between biological facts and social values. *American Psychologist, 47,* 373–88.

Wakefield, J. C. (1993). Limits of operationalization: a critique of Spitzer and Endicott's (1978) proposed operational criteria for mental disorder. *Journal of Abnormal Psychology, 102,* 160–72.

Wakefield, J. C. (1995). Dysfunction as a value-free concept: a reply to Sadler and Agich. *Philosophy, Psychiatry & Psychology, 2,* 233–46.

Wakefield, J. C. (1997). Diagnosing DSM-IV – Part I: DSM-IV and the concept of disorder. *Behaviour Research and Therapy, 35,* 633–49.

Wakefield, J. C. (1999a). Evolutionary versus prototype analysis of the concept of disorder. *Journal of Abnormal Psychology, 108,* 374–99.

Wakefield, J. C. (1999b). Mental disorder as a black box essentialist concept. *Journal of Abnormal Psychology, 108,* 465–72.

Wakefield, J. C. (2001). Evolutionary history versus current causal role in the definition of disorder: reply to McNally. *Behaviour Research and Therapy, 39,* 309–14.

Wakefield, J. C., Horwitz, A. V. & Schmitz, M. F. (2005). Are we over-pathologizing the socially anxious? Social phobia from a harmful dysfunction perspective. *Canadian Journal of Psychiatry, 50,* 317–19.

Walter, H. (2001). *Neurophilosophy of Free Will: From Libertarian Illusions to a Concept of Natural Autonomy* (translated by C. Klohr). Cambridge, MA: Bradford Books.

Walters, L. & Palmer, J. G. (1997). *The Ethics of Human Gene Therapy.* New York, NY: Oxford University Press.

Walton, S. (2004). *Humanity: An Emotional History.* London: Atlantic Books.

Wasson, R. G., Kramrisch, S., Ruck, S. & Ott, J. (1988). *Persephone's Quest: Entheogens and the Origins of Religion.* New Haven, CT: Yale University Press.

Watson, G. (2003). *Free Will.* Oxford: Oxford University Press.

Wegner, D. (2002). *The Illusion of Conscious Will.* Cambridge, MA: MIT Press.

Weisberger, A. M. (1995). The ethics of the broader usage of Prozac: social choice or social bias? *International Journal of Applied Philosophy*, **10**, 69–74.

Wells, K. B. (1999). Treatment research at the crossroads: the scientific interface of clinical trials and effectiveness research. *American Journal of Psychiatry*, **156**, 5–10.

Wexler, B. E. (2006). *Brain and Culture: Neurobiology, Ideology and Social Change.* Cambridge, MA: MIT Press.

Wheeler, M. (2005). *Reconstructing the Cognitive World.* Cambridge, MA: MIT Press.

White, L., Tursky, B. & Schwartz, G. E. (1985). *Placebo: Theory, Research, and Mechanisms.* New York, NY: Guilford.

White, S. L. (1991). *The Unity of the Self.* Cambridge, MA: MIT Press.

Whitehead, A. N. (1948). *Science and the Modern World.* New York, NY: New American Library.

Whitehouse, P. J., Juengst, E. Mehlman, M., *et al.* (1997). Enhancing cognition in the intellectually intact: possibilities and pitfalls. *Hastings Center Report*, **27**, 14–22.

Whiten, A. & Boesch, C. (2001). The cultures of chimpanzees. *Scientific American*, **284**, 60–7.

Wiggins, O. P. & Schwartz, M. A. (1991). Is there a science of meaning? *Integrative Psychiatry*, **1**, 48–53.

Wijsbeck, H. (2000). The pursuit of beauty: the enforcement of aethetics or a freely adopted lifestyle? *Journal of Medical Ethics*, **26**, 454–8.

Wilkes, K. (1988). *Real People: Personality Identity without Thought Experiments.* Oxford: Oxford University Press.

Willett, W. C. & Stampfer, M. J. (2001). What vitamins should I be taking, doctor? *New England Journal of Medicine*, **345**, 1819–24.

Williams, B. (1985). *Ethics and the Limits of Philosophy.* London: Fontana Press/Collins.

Williams, B. (1994). *Problems of the Self: Philosophical Papers 1956–1972.* Cambridge: Cambridge University Press.

Winch, P. (1970). *The Idea of a Social Science and its Relation to Philosophy.* Atlantic Highlands, NJ: Humanities Press.

Wing, J. K. (1978). *Reasoning about Madness.* Oxford: Oxford University Press.

Wittgenstein, L. (1960). *The Blue and Brown Books.* Oxford: Blackwell.

Wittgenstein, L. (1980). *Remarks on the Philosophy of Psychology,* Vol. I (edited by G. E. M. Anscombe & G. H. von Wright). Oxford: Blackwell.

Wittgenstein, L. (1982). Conversations on Freud. In R. Wollheim & J. Hopkins. *Philosophical Essays on Freud.* Cambridge: Cambridge University Press.

Wittgenstein, L. J. J. (1967). *Philosophical Investigations* (translated by G. E. M. Anscombe, 3rd edn). London: Blackwell.

Witz, A. (2000). Whose body matters? Feminist sociology and the corporeal turn in sociology and feminism. *Body & Society,* **6,** 1–24.

Wolfe, S. M. (2003). Ephedra – scientific evidence versus money/politics. *Science,* **300,** 437.

Wollheim, R. (1984). *The Thread of Life.* Cambridge, MA: Harvard University Press.

Wollheim, R. (1999). *On the Emotions.* New Haven, CT: Yale University Press.

Wollheim, R. & Hopkins, J. (1982). *Philosophical Essays on Freud.* Cambridge: Cambridge University Press.

Wolpe, P. (2002). Treatment, enhancement, and the ethics of neurotherapeutics. *Brain and Cognition,* **50,** 387–95.

Wright, L. (1976). *Teleological Explanation.* Berkeley, CA: University of California Press.

Wright, R. (1995). *The Moral Animal: Why We Are the Way We Are – The New Science of Evolutionary Psychology.* New York, NY: Vintage Books.

Yehuda, R. & McFarlane, A. C. (1995). Conflict between current knowledge about posttraumatic stress disorder and its original conceptual basis. *American Journal of Psychiatry,* **152,** 1705–13.

Young, A. (1995). *The Harmony of Illusions: Inventing Post-Traumatic Stress Disorder.* Princeton, NJ: Princeton University Press.

Zachar, P. (2000). *Psychological Concepts and Biological Psychiatry: A Philosophical Analysis.* Amsterdam: John Benjamins.

Zachar, P. & Kendler, K. S. (2007). Psychiatric disorders: a conceptual taxonomy. *American Journal of Psychiatry,* **164,** 557–65.

Zacharacopoulou, E. (2006). *Beyond the Mind–Body Dualism: Psycho-analysis and the Human Body.* Amsterdam: Elsevier.

Zaner, R. M. (1981). *The Context of Self: A Phenomenological Inquiry Using Medicine as a Clue.* Athens, OH: Ohio University Press.

Zaner, R. M. (1993). *Troubled Voices: Stories of Ethics and Illness.* Cleveland, OH: The Pilgrim Press.

Zohar, J., Insel, T. R. & Zohar-Kadouch, R. C. (1988). Serotonergic responsivity in obsessive–compulsive disorder: effects of chronic clomipramine treatment. *Archives of General Psychiatry,* **45**, 167–72.

Zola, I. K. (1972). Medicine as an institution of social control. *Sociological Review,* **20**, 487–504.

Index